Praise for *Being Single, w*

"I have known Tracy for more than a decade, and watched her overcome many challenges, including cancer. It is through our own struggles that we learn to seek the growth and development that is possible when we embrace, rather than resist, whatever comes our way. *Being Single, with Cancer* takes the reader on a spiritual journey that solidifies for them that they are not alone, they have options, they are lovable and loved, and further, that they are powerful, inspirational, and divine in their own right."

—Christine Hassler, author of *Expectation Hangover*, Life Coach, and Speaker

"After hearing the three scariest words in the English language—you have cancer—on three separate occasions in college, I learned how difficult it can be for young adults to navigate cancer, which is what led me to found the Ulman Cancer Fund for Young Adults, and what leads me to endorse *Being Single, with Cancer*. Like the Foundation, this book provides resources, support, guidance, and, most of all, hope for those who may feel alone in facing cancer."

—Doug Ulman, President and CEO, LIVESTRONG Foundation

"This book will make a huge difference to you when facing a cancer diagnosis. Tracy's experience led to creating more freedom, a deeper connection to spirit, and an abiding joy in her own life, and she tells you how to do the same. This book has life lessons for everyone, whether single or not, survivor or not. I urge you to read the book and add it to your library."

—Patrick Snow, internationally bestselling author of *Creating Your Own Destiny* and *The Affluent Entrepreneur*

"What inspires me the most about Tracy's journey is her clear approach to growth and empowerment. She knows herself deeply and she remains open to gaining more knowledge through inquiry, curiosity, and living life fully. She is a wise woman who has chosen to expand, share, teach and empower others by listening to her own call to help other single survivors find the light within them. Consider yourself blessed to have picked up this book."

—Wendy De Rosa, Founder, School of Intuitive Studies, and author of *Energy Healing Through the Chakras: A Guide to Self-Healing*

"This book takes the reader on a journey of a true survivor who took control of her own healing through diet, uncovering destructive patterns in her emotions, setting boundaries, and making her own health and well-being a priority. . ... This book will help you know for sure that no matter what, you are never alone and you are always loved."

—Nicole Gabriel, author of *Finding Your Inner Truth*

"I so wish I had this book when I was 'single with cancer.' It is so needed. Tracy has filled a void and will give hope to so many facing cancer alone. And what readers will find is that they are actually not alone. *Being Single, with Cancer* leaves no stone unturned."

—Tamika Felder Campbell, Founder, Tamika & Friends and Cervical Cancer Survivor

"If you want to learn how to overcome adversity with grace and admiration, read Tracy's book."

—**Marcia Donziger, Founder, MyLifeLine.Org, and Ovarian Cancer Survivor**

"When I was diagnosed with cancer I was also single, and quite frankly, it sucked. But if given the choice today, I'd likely choose Tracy Maxwell's healing advice over a boyfriend! Like a best friend, Tracy tells the truth and cuts to the core of what we really need to hear as single survivors empowered to heal our deepest wounds while we conquer cancer....Tracy Maxwell is a truth-teller who challenges us to look inside instead of outside for the deeper, more permanent healing solutions we seek."

—**Emily Hine, Writer, Speaker, and Peace Officer, HolySit.com**

"*Being Single, with Cancer* is a powerful story of a cancer diagnosis unexpectedly turning out to be a blessing. Tracy's story resonates with anyone facing difficult circumstances yet determined to fight their way through with an open heart."

—**Gina Marotta, Heart Healer and Truth Activator**

"*Being Single, with Cancer* is a powerful tool for single people facing cancer or other serious diseases. As a three-time cancer survivor and newlywed, I'm personally aware of the difficulties of being single with a history of cancer....Tracy's frank discussions and exercises are also very helpful for the single (and not-so-single) guys out there, though we might not be comfortable admitting it."

—**Jasan Zimmerman, Healthy Young Attitude Facilitator and Three-time Cancer Survivor**

"When you're facing a frightening new reality, you quickly discover how little you know about what's ahead. That makes you feel small, dumb, unprepared, and terrified. Gaining that knowledge leads to confidence, which leads to realistic preparation, which leads to faith, which leads to empowerment. Tracy knows this journey all too well, and reading her book will move you closer to empowerment so that you can spend less time stumbling and more time recovering."

—**T.J. Sullivan, Co-Founder and CEO, CAMPUSPEAK, and author of** *Motivating the Middle*

"All people really want to know—especially those living with a disease—is that others have experienced something similar and come out stronger on the other side. Living with cancer is lonely for anyone, but dealing with cancer while single can be exponentially more difficult. Tracy shares her struggles with her readers and, in the process, empowers them to keep pushing through...keep living, and even to see the blessings in their illness. It takes an amazing amount of vulnerability to share yourself like Tracy has, and she has done so for the benefit of others."

—**Mike Dilbeck, Founder and Speaker, RESPONSE ABILITY: The Revolution for Courageous Leadership**

Being Single, with Cancer

A Solo Survivor's Guide to Life, Love, Health, and Happiness

Tracy Maxwell

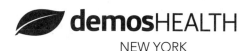

NEW YORK

Visit our website at www.demoshealth.com

ISBN: 978-1-936303-41-0
e-book ISBN: 978-1-617051-37-1

Acquisitions Editor: Julia Pastore
Compositor: diacriTech

Enough Manifesto graphics by Pamela Graglia

Medical information provided by Demos Health, in the absence of a visit with a health care professional, must be considered as an educational service only. This book is not designed to replace a physician's independent judgment about the appropriateness or risks of a procedure or therapy for a given patient. Our purpose is to provide you with information that will help you make your own health care decisions.

The information and opinions provided here are believed to be accurate and sound, based on the best judgment available to the authors, editors, and publisher, but readers who fail to consult appropriate health authorities assume the risk of injuries. The publisher is not responsible for errors or omissions. The editors and publisher welcome any reader to report to the publisher any discrepancies or inaccuracies noticed.

Library of Congress Cataloging-in-Publication Data

Maxwell, Tracy.
  Being single, with cancer: a solo survivor's guide to life, love, health, and happiness / Tracy Maxwell.
    pages cm
  Includes bibliographical references and index.
  ISBN 978-1-936303-41-0 — ISBN 978-1-61705-137-1 1. Cancer in women—Popular works.
2. Cancer in women—Psychological aspects—Popular works. I. Title.
  RC281.W65M27 2014
  616.99'40082—dc23
                                   2014010895

Special discounts on bulk quantities of Demos Health books are available to corporations, professional associations, pharmaceutical companies, health care organizations, and other qualifying groups. For details, please contact:

Special Sales Department
Demos Medical Publishing, LLC
11 West 42nd Street, 15th Floor
New York, NY 10036
Phone: 800-532-8663 or 212-683-0072
Fax: 212-941-7842
E-mail: specialsales@demosmedical.com

Printed in the United States of America by McNaughton & Gunn.
14 15 16 17 18 / 5 4 3 2 1

*This book is dedicated to Alli Ward. Helping her live
her life fully in the face of death
showed me the value I could provide to others
if I too were willing to take the risk.*

Contents

A New Beginning

You are alone because you've decided you are unlovable, unworthy, and unappreciated. You are damaged goods and no one could possibly ever want you. Your beliefs are killing you, and they created cancer in your body. You are single, and you will always be single. No one is ever going to love you.

I understand how you feel. I've had these same thoughts.

Are you concerned about how to tell a potential love interest that you've had cancer?

Are you infertile as a result of your treatment?

Are you afraid the cancer might come back?

Are you discouraged about life?

Are you concerned about the costs of medical treatment?

Do you wonder who will take care of you?

Are you worried you might die from this?

I've asked myself these questions, too. I know what it is like to lie in bed at night, alone and scared, and wonder if it is ever going to be OK. I have questioned if something is wrong with me that I am in my forties and still single. I have doubted that anyone would want me with surgery scars, missing body parts, infertility, and the looming threat of recurrence hanging over my head. I know what it is like to be a single cancer survivor.

In this book, you will hear from single survivors like yourself who will share their fears, triumphs, and disappointments. You will know for sure that you are not alone, and that you have options for treating your cancer and living your life more fully. You will learn to take responsibility for your life, and even to embrace your survivor status. You will complete exercises to help you take control and create the kind of inspirational, powerful, and loving life that you deserve. You will recognize your own value, worth, and uniqueness, and discover how you can share your special gifts with the world. Most of all, you will get that you are truly and completely loved and lovable.

I invite you to read it as a personal letter from me to you about what I wish I had known when I began my own journey, and what I learned along the way. *Being Single, with Cancer* provides tips for navigating through each stage of your journey from diagnosis and treatment through survivorship and life beyond cancer. It addresses getting the support you need and managing the emotional impacts, and it insists that you take responsibility for your own care and own your power through the process.

It includes my personal experience, interviews with several solo survivors, and results from a survey I conducted with approximately 100 cancer survivors from across the United States. I was thrilled at how many people were so willing to share their stories so openly and allow me to use their names in the book. Mostly, I use only first names, and in a couple of cases I have changed names as requested. By reading the experiences of single survivors, I hope you will feel less alone and more empowered.

The survey results weren't surprising. The issues that floated to the top included: Dating anxiety, body image, loneliness, fertility problems, and a desire for more support. Some reported serious financial issues, lack of health insurance, and having to move back in with their parents for help. A significant number shared how overwhelmed they felt having to make so many huge decisions on their own. Many of those I interviewed now feel called to help others through sharing their stories, starting a nonprofit, volunteering, raising money for the cancer community, or all of the above.

Most of the well-known organizations founded to serve young adult cancer survivors were started by, and many continue to be run by, single people. Whether seeking to fill a void in our lives, or simply free from distractions posed by spouses and families, it is interesting that singles have played a major role in reaching out to help others through this experience.

Single young adult survivors also seem to be more connected to support services, perhaps because we find ourselves in need of more support. Camps, conferences, adventure programs, and even mentoring programs appear to have more single participants. One year, 95 percent of participants in First Descents outdoor adventure programs were single!

The experiences shared in the book come from a wide variety of perspectives. Some of the survivors interviewed had also lost parents to cancer, and others had just left marriages or long-term relationships when their cancer struck. One signed divorce papers from the hospital. Another left her husband with $20 in her pocket, nowhere to live, no car, no job, no health insurance, and two small children, only to be diagnosed with ovarian cancer two weeks later. A third left a relationship of 16 years in January, lost his dad in March, and in June was diagnosed with esophageal cancer. In the two years this book has been in progress, several of the survivors interviewed have gotten engaged or married, including Tamika, Jasan, Leah, and Heather.

I wrote this book because I've been where you are. I've been afraid and felt so alone that I didn't know if life was even worth living. Cancer gave me the wake up call I needed to face my fears and take responsibility for my life. It was the catalyst for embracing my community, asking for their help, and gratefully receiving what they had to offer, including emotional and financial support, wisdom and information, physical care taking, inspiration, and so much more love than I ever could have imagined. As a speaker, author, blogger, facilitator, coach, and part-time river guide, I have the good fortune to share what I've learned with so many people, and I feel so blessed to do so.

As I have navigated the ins and outs of living with disease over the past several years, I have realized that while the physical issues were considerable, my biggest challenges were emotional, and that being single played a large role in my experience, in how I saw things, in how I dealt with my illness and what I learned about myself and my life. I began blogging about life as a single survivor on my one-year cancerversary (the anniversary of my diagnosis), but little did I know then that my journey wasn't over and my cancer would return twice more.

It began with serious stomach pain on New Year's Day 2006 that landed me in the emergency room in the middle of the night, with what I was told at the time was a harmless ovarian cyst that had burst. Instructed to follow up with my gynecologist, we soon discovered that the cyst had returned, and after watching it for a few months, my doctor finally decided surgery was required. Though the surgery went well, there were no complications, and I was sent home immediately from the outpatient procedure, I knew it wasn't going to be good news when I got a call to come in the next day to discuss the pathology of the mass they removed.

After another more invasive surgery in which my right ovary was removed and I spent three days in the hospital, I received the diagnosis of stage IIc granulosa cell ovarian cancer. A medical oncologist was assigned and six rounds of chemo prescribed. Following that, a hysterectomy was recommended, second opinions gathered, and a decision to hold on to my "girl parts" as long as possible was made. Eventually, I did give them up when three new spots showed up on an ultrasound in 2010.

Rather than do more chemo, following my now third surgery I radically changed my diet and began taking a more holistic approach to my health that included supplements, emotional and energy work, chiropractic, naturopathy, and Chinese medicine. That didn't keep the cancer at bay though, and in December of 2011 two new masses were detected on a follow-up scan. These were bigger than before, and they grew somewhat steadily as my blood counts rose over the course of the next year.

More surgery was debated, but my surgeon expressed reluctance to expose me to the risks of surgery every time something new showed up, since it appeared this could be a regular occurrence. In December of 2012, four new smaller masses popped up where my ovaries used to be, and after six months of watching them grow, it was finally decided that surgery was required when one of the masses began pushing against a kidney.

In July 2013, a grapefruit-size tumor and several smaller ones were removed from my abdomen. After a few weeks of recovery, I traveled to California to work with an alternative cancer clinic that utilized a number of natural therapies, in hopes of keeping the cancer from returning. I also spent a week at a nutritional detox program that involved a mind–body–spirit approach, and pursued emotional and energetic healing techniques through these clinics and outside of them.

I don't know what the future holds for me in terms of this disease. I have the type of cancer that isn't cured after a five-year remission rate. On the positive side, it's not aggressive, so we are likely to always spot it in time to treat, but on the downside, it could come back anytime, even as many as 30 years later. Given that I have already had two recurrences in seven years, this seems more likely than not. I do know this: I may have cancer, but cancer doesn't have me. Since 2010, I have not lived my life as a cancer patient. I complete my follow-up visits as scheduled and take responsibility for my health, but I don't worry about what is going on in there. I believe that I am healed, and I feel great. Even with a grapefruit-sized mass in my abdomen, I didn't experience pain, fatigue, or concern. I am at peace about whatever happens next, and absolutely know that I am going to be OK—that I AM OK.

I know it is not always easy for everyone to feel the way I do. For some, a follow-up scan causes major anxiety, and the fear is always there that the cancer could return, that it could be untreatable, and that you will have to face it alone again. I know that being a cancer patient can feel like a full-time job. I know that you might be thinking I'm crazy for feeling the way I do. At times I have felt completely overwhelmed with the amount of time, energy, and money it takes to eat healthy, juice, meditate, exercise regularly, date, spend time with friends and family, pursue alternative treatments that aren't covered by health insurance and, oh, maintain a career that allows me to do all those things.

Cancer is stressful in the extreme, and facing it alone can make you wonder if it's all worth it. I don't want you to beat yourself up if you haven't managed to be peaceful in the face of disease; if you don't eat as healthy as you want to, get as much sleep as you require, or own a juicer; if exercise is something you wish you could find time and energy for; if dating and meditating seem like pipe dreams. It's OK.

Cancer is never easy, and dealing with a serious illness as a single person is a unique experience. Our ranks are growing as cancer strikes at younger ages, many of us put off marriage until later, and the aging population loses spouses to death or divorce. Fifty percent of American adults are single, and 31 million (1 in 7) of us live alone, according to the book *Going Solo*. People who live alone make up 28 percent of all U.S. households, making them even more common than those containing a nuclear family.

While there are a multitude of resources for cancer patients, there is nothing specifically for those of us who are single. Because of this lack of resources, I have long been interested in supporting solo survivors, and I started an organization to do so. I want to be your guide, to share with you what I've learned over eight years and three rounds of cancer. I want to support you on your journey so you will absolutely know you are never alone! It is one of the greatest joys of my life to coach people in discovering the truth of who they really are, and helping them find joy and peace and purpose in their lives.

So, are you ready to begin? I am going to ask you to forget everything you thought you knew about cancer, and about what it means to be single. This book will require you to step out of your comfort zone, stretch your mind, and open yourself to new possibilities. You will be challenged to consider new ways of thinking about who you are, how much you are loved and supported, and what you have to offer to the world. Though you may be tempted to skip over the exercises to keep reading the content, I encourage you to give yourself the gift of the insights each exercise can provide, and to recognize that doing them in order when they appear will set you up for receiving the most out of what comes next. I am so excited to help you discover the real you, the authentic and beautiful you, the healed and healthy and lovable and loved YOU! Let's go!

ONE

Diagnosis and Treatment

CHAPTER

1

You Are Not Alone

We're born alone, we live alone, we die alone.
Only through our love and friendship
can we create the illusion for the moment that we're not alone.
—ORSON WELLES

It's often just enough to be with someone.
I don't need to touch them. Not even talk.
A feeling passes between you both. You're not alone.
—MARILYN MONROE

Feeling *alone* is far worse than having cancer.

This is what many survivors told me, and what I instinctively know myself.

Most of the time I am very satisfied, even ecstatic, with my life as an independent, single woman. My lifestyle allows me to do the things I want to do when I want to do them. If I feel like staying in bed all day on a cold, rainy Sunday afternoon reading a book, I can do it. When I want to jump in my car or hop on a plane for a fun weekend getaway, only my budget might prevent me. I don't have to pick up someone else's dirty socks or put the toilet seat down constantly or put up with annoying in-laws. I can go wherever I want on vacation, spend holidays with my family, and paint the living room any color I like. There are no demands from a partner or children that get in the way of my needs. I feel lucky to live in a time and culture that allows me the freedom to live independently, and I make the most of that freedom to live the kind of life that I want to live.

Most days, being single is pretty OK if not downright great. But when things are at their worst, when I'm sick or struggling with a household problem, or just having a garden variety bad day, I feel really alone because I don't have a partner to help out or comfort me. I think: I will always be alone, and I will have only myself to rely on. I fantasize about how much easier it would be if I had a partner. Financial hardship wouldn't be so bad with another income to fall back on. Health scares would be easier with someone there to hold my hand or give me a hug.

One 29-year-old female survivor said, "I've always hated how society makes such a big deal about being single, like it's so pathetic how your self-worth is tied to that. I never felt that way, aside from occasional loneliness, I could function just fine and was happy," she said. "Getting cancer was another story, though. Without a strong support network, it was difficult, and I had to admit for the first time that my single status was a detriment."

Another survey participant volunteered, "I realized how alone I was when hit with such a serious life event. My siblings and parents are halfway across the country, and my friends all work, so they weren't always available."

I know that not all partnerships are happy all the time, and that many a serious diagnosis has also been followed soon thereafter by breakup or divorce. I also know it is better to be single than to be in a relationship where I don't feel supported or cared for. Intellectually, I know that the grass is not always greener, but sometimes it feels like it is.

I assume that dealing with cancer would be more endurable with someone who loves me by my side—someone to hold me in the middle of the night when I'm afraid; someone to be there for every doctor appointment and procedure; someone to tell me it's going to be OK when it just doesn't seem like it ever will again. Married friends who have been diagnosed, or even those who have dealt with a serious health issue or accident, have marveled at how I did it on my own.

Other single survivors who were surveyed expressed similar feelings. "What was most lacking for me was companionship. I went to treatment and doctors alone, and it was hard to remember all the important information, and lonely being surrounded by others who were there with loved ones."

Another shared, "The loneliness was sometimes unbearable. Friends help some, but it's not the same as having a partner." Someone else offered,

"I often felt alone during treatment—for a significant other, that is. It's hard to admit, but after an experience like that, I often worry that I will not find a person that I could spend my life with and that it could be too late."

Of course, everyone goes through cancer alone. No one else can ever really understand what the experience is like, and it's unique for each person. But as a single person, I've felt a special type of alone: devastatingly alone. There is so much to learn, so much to do and so many decisions to make about doctors, treatment options, financial considerations, and it can feel so overwhelming to make those by myself. It is one thing to have lots of great friends to support you (and I am lucky that I do), but it's not a substitute for having one person who loves you unconditionally by your side.

"I felt so lonely," said one survey participant. "Friends and family can't understand what you are going through and aren't there when you have insomnia and the loneliness hits hard. It would be nice if there were support groups for single young people."

Another added, "Nights were the hardest. It was the time I was left alone with my thoughts, which were tough to deal with."

When I spiral, my friends remind me that I may not have a partner but I am not alone. I am part of a community that cares for me, and friends and family have always provided support when I needed it. Within the first hour of my most recent health crisis, three people in my life dropped what they were doing to come to my aid. Those loving relationships are just as important and essential as any committed partner, yet my feeling of aloneness often persists. Through my survey, I've realized this is common for single cancer survivors. Nearly 80 percent of the 100 single cancer survivors I interviewed reported feeling alone, and 77 percent cited connections with other cancer survivors as a top need.

Survey participants shared the following thoughts:

"Feeling isolated with my illness fed depression, which just made everything worse."

───────────────◦◦───────────────

"Feeling alone sucked. I had no one my age who could relate to what I was going through."

───────────────◦◦───────────────

"Even though I have a large support network, being without a partner was hard when it came to making treatment decisions. The nighttime is the toughest to be alone."

───────────────◦◦───────────────

The idea that if you haven't found "the one" then you are missing the only thing that really matters is also common. As one woman said, "I often don't feel I have much to live and fight for. So many times you hear people battling cancer say things like, 'If it weren't for wanting to be with my spouse, I don't know how I could have done it all.' Or people want to survive to be there for their children. If my life ended, it wouldn't really be a big deal to anyone but my mom, so motivation is pretty hard to come by when you're faced with side effects, stress, anxiety, bad news, uncomfortable tests, horrid procedures, putting your life on hold, debt, and never having any time or money or energy. And all for what?"

When do you feel most alone?

With whom can you share what you are going through?

What makes you feel the most connected to others?

The Importance of Connection

Since you cannot do good to all, you are to pay special attention to those who, by the accidents of time, or place, or circumstances, are brought into closer connection with you.
—SAINT AUGUSTINE

I've had moments when I've thought about somebody, picked up the phone to call them and they are on the line already, and I think that maybe there's some vibration, some connection.
—CLINT EASTWOOD

Feeling alone is one of the most destructive emotions we can have. Research has shown that loneliness can impact stress, health, and immunity. According to Dr. Dean Ornish in his book *Love & Survival*, "Our survival depends on the healing power of love, intimacy, and relationships." When we lack those connections, we suffer. He cites numerous studies about the key role played by family, friends, spouses, and social connections such as church/synagogue or other community associations in fighting illness. Lissa Rankin, MD, cites some of the same studies as well as others in her book *Mind Over Medicine: Scientific Proof That You Can Heal Yourself.*

If you are single and battling cancer or some other illness, connecting with the people in your life, or finding new sources of support, may be one of the most important things you can do for yourself. Ask for what

Sources of Support

In a survey of 100 single survivors, these were the most common sources of support:

- 50% family (survivors cited them as really helpful)
- 37% friends
- 35% church community
- 31% coworkers (the latter three were cited as somewhat helpful)

Half of the participants cited that romantic partners barely acknowledged what they were going through and weren't a major source of support, though most were not serious relationships.

you need. Whether it's talking on the phone more regularly, going out for a walk, sharing coffee once a week, visiting or hosting a friend or sibling for a weekend, joining a support group, participating in group meditation or yoga classes, serving others directly, or any number of other things, do what you can to connect with the world around you.

It turns out that being single can be a predictor of shorter survival times and an increased chance of recurrence. And the studies don't just relate to cancer patients. In fact, Ornish's work is primarily with heart disease, but the findings suggest that even the common cold can be better protected against with quality social networks and interaction.

The most striking study cited was conducted by Dr. David Spiegel and colleagues at Stanford in 1989. Published in the British journal *The Lancet*, they studied women with metastatic breast cancer. Spiegel initially set out to prove that social connection did not have an impact on survival. Participants in the study were divided into two groups—both of which received the same conventional treatments such as chemotherapy, radiation, and surgery. One group also met together for 90 minutes each week over the course of a year to talk about the impact of the disease on their lives. They became comfortable enough to share their feelings openly, including fears of disfigurement, abandonment, and even death.

Five years later, Dr. Spiegel reviewed the data and was shocked to discover that women in the support group lived on average twice as long as the control group, and that all of the women in the group without support had since died. Dr. Spiegel wrote the book *Living Beyond Limits* about the extraordinary findings of this study. Other studies have shown that support groups as short as six weeks long have had similar outcomes for the people who attended regularly. Each study controlled for diet, exercise, family history, and other factors that typically impact disease, and found significant advantages to social connection even beyond these other factors.

Do the statistics mean that those of us who are single are doomed to get sick more often and die sooner than our married or partnered friends? Absolutely not! In fact, marriages with problems—a great deal of disagreement or stress—have been shown to produce negative effects as well. Support can come in many forms: a close network of friends with whom you can share your fears, a support group of other people who understand what you are going through, a close family, or strong ties to a religious or other community. No matter what form it takes, it requires a willingness to be vulnerable enough to truly open yourself up to others.

That last factor is perhaps the most difficult for many of us, and yet, the most important to truly offer authentic connection. It isn't the quantity of support that matters, but the quality. In other words, it's not the number of people who are there for you that counts, but how connected you feel with those who are around, and how much you can truly share what you are dealing with.

Sage Advice

From Sage Bolte, PhD, LCSW, OSW-C, oncology counselor and social worker

- Don't try to do it alone. Ask for help. People want to help and don't perceive it as a burden.
- Get creative to broaden your support system. Not just family, but also friends, church, or other survivors.
- Talk about your experiences both inside and outside of cancer.
- Work with a therapist if you find that cancer is defining who you are, rather than being a part of your story.

Dr. Bolte recommends four associations to help you find a qualified therapist. You can find these listed in the resources section under Counselors and Therapists.

Support Groups

Interestingly, more of the men I interviewed participated in support groups than women. Jeremie said about his medical team, "I was really impressed with the level of caring I received from my health care providers. I have a much greater appreciation for what they do. They were genuinely concerned and go above and beyond. I had no bad experiences throughout that whole thing."

Jeremie was impressed by all the services provided by his cancer center in Minnesota as well, and found out about a support group from his surgeon. It meets once a month and is run by a nurse practitioner and a psychologist. He is the youngest guy in the group, but was happy to find two other guys there who were not only close to his age, but also recovering alcoholics like him. Having multiple things in common with other group members was important to him. It wasn't just about cancer.

"I'm almost more proud of the fact that I didn't get hooked on any of the drugs that I was put on during cancer treatment," he said. "My addictive personality led me down this road again, so when the pain started to go away, I weaned myself off the drugs or I knew I would never get back to normal. One day I just threw it all out and that was that. Now I don't even take Tylenol. That was a big turning point for me. It would have been easy to get drugs as a cancer patient."

Jasan, a three-time cancer survivor, has regularly attended a support group for young adults for more than 10 years now. He read an article in the paper about the Bay Area group and felt compelled to go. Though he didn't talk at all the first year, sharing only his name and diagnosis, he slowly became more comfortable. Finally being around a positive, safe environment helped, he said.

"I'm a typical dude that doesn't want to talk about my feelings," he said. "My mom would always try to get me to talk about it, but I never wanted to. Now I know there is freedom in talking about it. It really makes me feel good that I can help other people by sharing my own experience."

The majority of single survivors I interviewed for this book did not report participation in a support group. Some of them, like me, found them to be more depressing than helpful, and couldn't relate to the mostly elderly group members in far different stages of life. Those who found a group of people their age with similar issues and concerns, however, reported significant benefits.

How socially connected are you? What are some of the groups mentioned that you interact with regularly?

What kind of support group or social network would appeal to you? How might you find such a community?

What are some ways you could connect more fully with your existing communities?

The book *Going Solo* suggests that singles who live in urban areas are actually more socially connected than their married counterparts, largely because the latter interact primarily with each other, while singles in cities get out more with others in social settings. This kind of connection with others, whether they have cancer or not, can also be beneficial.

Other factors that have been proven to influence healing and well-being according to Ornish:

* Roommates or living with family
* Pets
* Touch—massage, Reiki, or just holding the hand of a friend
* Community involvement and service
* Yoga and meditation (or other relaxation techniques)

Pets and Single Survivors

I have often heard the advice that if you are single, you should have a pet, since they provide a motivation to get up in the morning, get home at a reasonable hour from work, and even help promote exercise, all in service to your pet's needs. Though my travel schedule and small condo have been deterrents for me in this area, I think it is great advice. I often say that while I don't have my own, I love other people's kids and pets.

Jeremie shared that although women have come and gone from his life, his dog is a constant source of companionship and love. "I am always hugging and squeezing her," he said. A beagle–bluetick mix, she was a stray that his ex-girlfriend just brought home one day. "No one knew where she came from," he said "but I don't know what I would have done without her. I honestly believe she is one of the loves of my life."

Susan felt the same way about Kaya, her Great Dane who turned into a protector practically overnight when Susan was diagnosed with ovarian cancer. Kaya could sense when Susan was having physical problems. Adopted when she was just one year old, Susan's huge dog was destructive, nervous, and suffering from serious separation anxiety when she first came home.

In January of 2010, Susan had major surgery and received her diagnosis. She says almost immediately a new side of Kaya's personality emerged. When Susan came home following surgery, her four-legged friend was elated, but sensed a need to be gentle as she quietly sniffed Susan from head to toe.

"When she reached my incision area (a 12-inch vertical slash across my abdomen), she stopped sniffing and looked up at me with a worried expression," Susan said. "She was very sweet and gentle, which is saying a lot because she's a bit of a lug. Kaya is many things, but graceful is not one of them."

The day after arriving home from the hospital, Susan's friend came to stay with her to help with her recovery. As Susan moved from the couch to the bedroom, her friend got up to follow her and Kaya began to growl, backing the friend into a corner and not allowing her near Susan. "I was shocked," Susan said. "In the three years since I had adopted her, I had NEVER heard her growl."

Susan described typical Kaya behavior as: running for the hills at the sight of a bug, hiding in the bedroom when someone was at the front door, and snacking on the couch until it was unrecognizable. Susan went on to describe her laughter at the call from doggie day care once informing her that Kaya had to be moved to the small dog room because she was being bullied by a German shepherd.

"I know it's weird (and inappropriate) to be proud about a dog growling at another person," Susan says, "but it felt good to know that she was protecting the 'injured' member of her pack, and the hockey player in me was happy to see her assert herself a little."

Kaya took her guardian role very seriously throughout Susan's recovery. When daily injections of blood thinner into Susan's stomach were required during the first week, and the shots left her with tears streaming down her face, Kaya tried to protect her from this pain by standing between the bed and the person with the shot.

Kaya got even more protective when Susan started chemotherapy. Sniffing her head to toe when she returned home following the first infusion, Susan believes she could smell the chemicals in her system. "During the days and weeks that I was recovering from chemo, Kaya literally would not leave my side," she says. "My mom and friends would have to coax her off my bed in order to eat or go outside. She would lie quietly with me for hours and hours when I was not feeling well. If I slept, she slept. If I lay awake, she would peer into my eyes with a concerned care."

Once, when Susan was really sick, and another time before she was hospitalized with a serious fever, Kaya woke Susan's mom up in the middle of the night to check on the patient. Both times, Susan was sleeping soundly, but within 30 minutes began experiencing symptoms. Both Susan and her mom feel that Kaya sensed something was wrong and was trying to help. Though Kaya has since passed away, Susan is grateful that she was with her throughout her cancer treatment, and she continues to foster other Great Danes.

Your Circle Is Wider Than You Think

What should young people do with their lives today?
Many things, obviously.
But the most daring thing is to create stable communities in which
the terrible disease of loneliness can be cured.
—KURT VONNEGUT

You are part of a community. Several actually. We all are. There are those with whom we talk about books or movies, those we go hiking or biking with, those with whom we love to just hang out, those we love to eat out or cook with, those we know from a particular place such as church or school, those we see regularly, and those we only connect with virtually or talk with on the phone occasionally.

Try This

Take Stock of All the People in Your Life

Take out a journal, notebook, or even a poster board and begin to make a list or mind map of the communities you belong to. Your family is one. Your friends, another. You can create communities by era (high school, college, etc.) or areas of your life (work, school, hobbies, those who live near you, those who live far away, those you have lost touch with, those you see every day, those you miss) or whatever system that works for you. Include acquaintances, coworkers, role models, anyone who you know personally; they should all go on the list, even if you haven't connected with or seen them in a long time.

I am always amazed at how huge my list is, and it's never actually exhaustive. Some of my communities include: high school, college, sorority, camp, work, professional, graduate school, church, cancer, outdoor enthusiasts, writers, friends of friends, book club, family, river guides, and various pen pals through the years. Many people appear on several different lists and I keep adding to it as I make new connections and I remember people I haven't thought of in years.

Why is it useful to write down the people you know and the various communities they fall into? Because you don't really realize how many people are indeed in your life. You are surrounded by people who love you. Seeing it in black and white (or better yet, full color) will make it more real for you, and give you a resource to turn to when you are feeling alone.

What does community mean to you?

How has community impacted your life up to this point?

Try This

Connect with Three to Five People Each Day or Week

It's OK to text, e-mail, or Facebook message, but use a variety of methods to connect, including phone calls and face to face.

How many different people can you connect with this week? This month?

Keep a running tally and have some fun with it! Don't have an agenda for your connections? Just reach out. If something occurs to you to ask for, then do so. If help is offered, take it.

The Cancer Community

I refuse to join any club that would have me as a member.
—GROUCHO MARX

*Communication leads to community, that is,
to understanding, intimacy and mutual valuing.*
—ROLLO MAY

Like it or not, once you have been diagnosed with cancer, you become part of a club. It's not as exclusive as it used to be, unfortunately, but it can become a community if you choose. You listed the communities you belong to, and after you have been dealing with cancer for a while, fellow survivors that you come into contact with can make up a new category as well. Whether you meet them at a retreat, in a support group, or at the doctor's office, these fellow travelers can become an important part of your tribe. They get it. They have been there, and they are typically up on the latest cancer news. Thinking about a holistic approach? Your cancer buds probably know something about that. Looking to get into a clinical trial, ask a fellow survivor. Looking for a second opinion or a good book on a cancer-related topic, they can point you in the right direction.

All the personal stories I'm sharing in this book came from my cancer posse in some way. Either I knew them personally, or they were connected to me through someone I had met along the way. Jonny Imerman of Imerman Angels connected me to a number of single survivors. Some research conducted by the LIVESTRONG Young Adult Alliance (now called Critical Mass) a few years ago showed that Jonny was the best connected in that community, and anyone who has ever met him is not surprised to hear that. In his signature black Imerman Angels t-shirt and jeans, and with his shiny bald head, Jonny is easy to spot in a crowd, but it is his exuberant personality that he is really known for.

I first met Jonny in 2008 at the LIVESTRONG Summit in Columbus, Ohio. He came in for a hug and flashed me his megawatt smile. Talking with Jonny gives you the feeling you're the only person on the planet as he stands close, never breaks eye contact, and often maintains physical connection throughout the conversation. Jonny never forgets a name, and typically remembers the diagnosis as well. For years he would tell me I was still the only granulosa cell ovarian cancer survivor in the Imerman Angels database.

Jonny has been such a force in my survivorship, advising me early on about health insurance issues and taking time out of his busy schedule to talk on the phone or meet me for dinner when I'm in Chicago. He has been instrumental in the lives of so many others as well. His organization pairs cancer "fighters," those newly diagnosed, with cancer survivors like me who have been through the process of treatment and recovery. This mentorship provides an amazing opportunity to talk with someone who has been there and done that, and can share information and hope. Jonny truly believes these mentors are like angels to the freshly diagnosed when they are in the midst of so much fear and turmoil.

The idea for the organization grew out of his own experience of talking with other cancer patients in the hospital. "My room was always filled with family members and close friends," he said, "but in many other rooms, I saw people fighting cancer alone, lying in bed motionless, watching television or staring into space." He said he felt guilty at his abundance of support and positive energy, and vowed that if he was given a life after cancer, he would use it to help others.

I also experienced the power of the cancer community through First Descents, a nonprofit that brings together young adult cancer survivors for a week of adventure in some of the most beautiful settings in the world. One of my fellow campers said it best: "This is a cancer camp that's not about cancer." While we all knew we shared a cancer background and talked about it informally throughout our time together, it was never the focus. Enjoying each other, the great outdoors, and the challenge of a great adventure were the cornerstones of this experience.

The most beautiful gift of this program for many is simply being taken away from the grind of daily life to experience equal measures of tranquility, friendship, and adventure in a stunning natural setting. As our staff on the Montana kayaking adventure reminded us before our graduation paddle, we have only right here and right now. When you are paddling a class III rapid called Bone Crusher, or trying to avoid Can Opener Rock, cancer is the furthest thing from your mind. I am so grateful to have had this experience, and that nonprofits like First Descents exist to challenge and support us through this journey.

These are just two examples of the programs, resources, and support systems where everyone can find community in the cancer world. There

---

There are a number of incredible resources for cancer survivors, from those offering Reiki and massage, retreats and camps, financial support, or granting of wishes to the terminally ill, and just about everything in-between. If you have a need, the organization or program to fulfill it likely exists. Whether you are looking for a support group, a cancer mentor, a way to raise money and support a cause you care about, or coaching, a quick Internet search should yield a variety of resources. There is a long list at the end of this book, but new ones are popping up daily. Most of the organizations and programs will provide links to other services as well, so look for resources on every website. Many programs are national or global in scope, while others exist in your local community or through your hospital or doctor's office. Ask what is available, and speak to a social worker about options for you.

are programs for young adults (more and more all the time), teens, families, groups differentiated by gender, specific cancer types, and geography. There are active outdoor opportunities, quiet meditative retreats, strictly educational conferences and programs, and everything in-between. Check out the resources section for some ideas and search the Internet for a variety of other opportunities that meet your specific needs.

Whether you listen to the Stupid Cancer radio show for young adults, attend a retreat put on by Camp Mak-A-Dream, or learn to surf with Athletes for Cancer, I encourage you to find a way to get involved with your new community. It will help to connect with others who understand, and will definitely help you feel less alone.

Brian, a 32-year-old stage IV, non-Hodgkin's lymphoma survivor, used several services for cancer survivors from First Descents to Imerman Angels and Gilda's Club. He attended Stupid Cancer's OMG Conference and found it as well as their website and radio show extremely helpful. He also felt fortunate that a counselor he saw as a child reached out to him when he was diagnosed and offered to treat him for free; in addition, he and his younger brother, who is also a survivor, joined a support group for young adults that has been immensely helpful as well.

Heather Hall is an osteosarcoma survivor who works for Gilda's Club. She attended a session at Camp Mak-A-Dream a few years after her diagnosis. "Going there really made me realize there were others like me," she said. "The biggest thing is that you're NOT alone. There are so many resources. It is great to connect with others who are dealing with this."

What role would you like your new cancer community to play in your recovery?

What types of programs appeal to you? Active, outdoors, informational conferences, or small group retreats?

Imerman Angels is a one-to-one mentoring program matching newly diagnosed cancer patients or caregivers—"cancer fighters"—with those who have been through the same type of situation—"cancer survivors." People are matched with others who are similar to them on a variety of points—diagnosis, gender, age, geographic location, even religion, if that is noted as important.

(continued)

(*continued*)

> **Gilda's Club**, founded in honor of comedian Gilda Radner, who died of ovarian cancer in 1989, offers social and emotional support for cancer survivors and their families at a variety of clubhouses in cities across the United States.
>
> **Stupid Cancer** is a nonprofit organization that empowers young adults affected by cancer through innovative and award-winning programs and services. They are the nation's largest support community for this underserved population and serve as a bullhorn for the young adult cancer movement.
>
> **Camp Mak-A-Dream** provides medically supervised, cost-free Montana experiences, in an intimate community setting, for children, young adults, and families affected by cancer.
>
> Find more information about these resources and a variety of others in the back of the book.

Help Is Out There—If You Ask

Asking is the beginning of receiving. Make sure you don't go to the ocean with a teaspoon. At least take a bucket so the kids won't laugh at you.
—JIM ROHN

I think that the most difficult thing is allowing yourself to be loved, so receiving the love and feeling like you deserve it is a pretty big struggle. I suppose that's what I've learnt recently, to allow myself to be loved.
—NICOLE KIDMAN

Learning how to ask for help is one of the most valuable lessons I've learned from my cancer diagnosis. I was never good at asking for help, preferring to be a fiercely independent and self-sufficient person. Asking felt uncomfortable to me. It felt like a weaker position. What if the person I ask says "no"?

When I received a new TV for Christmas one year and faced the task of getting it into my house after driving with it for eight hours, I chose to carry it by inches rather than ask someone to help. When I broke my ankle, I was insistent upon being my typical independent, strong, and capable self, so I rarely let anyone see how hard that time was for me. I expected people to intuitively know I needed them, and what I needed, and come rushing over to provide it, and when they didn't, I was bitter. I spent a lot of time feeling sorry for myself, and complaining, but did a very poor job of explaining to people what I was going through. Had I been willing to admit that I was feeling down and lonely and helpless, I have no doubt my friends and family would have shown up for me in incredible ways to help me through it.

My friend Jenifer Madson's book *Living the Promises*, states: "We are never at a loss for support; only the words sometimes to ask for it." I was always surrounded by love and support, but I didn't know how to ask for what I needed or how to receive it when it was offered, until I got cancer.

Try This

Get the Support You Need

1. Take stock of all the people in your life. (You did this already with your communities.)
2. Figure out what you need.
3. Ask for help.
4. Keep people in the loop and be open about your challenges.
5. Receive graciously and gratefully.

When I got cancer, things were different. In many ways, having cancer was much easier than having a broken ankle. Even though I didn't feel well from the treatments much of the time, I still had full use of my body and people immediately wanted to know what they could do to help. My initial answer was, "I don't know." It was so new, and I didn't yet fully understand what impact this disease would have on my life.

I did know from experience that if I wanted help, I'd better figure out what it was that I needed and tell people. I decided to be completely transparent this time around, and really share what I was going through both physically and emotionally. I began posting regularly on a health website about the latest test results, treatment protocols, and emotional hurdles I was dealing with. I probably shared way more than I needed to, but it was cathartic for me.

Try This

Keep Friends and Family Updated On Your Condition and Needs

Use a service like Carepages, Caring Bridge, or Facebook. My favorite is MyLifeLine.org. This nonprofit site allows patients to share not just in a journal format and upload of photos, but also provides a treatment calendar, inspirational quotes, medical information, and a donation function to support the patient. It is just for cancer, and allows users to keep information private (to only those you invite or allow) or public to connect with other patients and survivors.

A service like this significantly cuts down on the number of times you have to repeat information, and makes it easy for loved ones to get updates. Keeping health and medical information separate from social media might be preferable to some. You have to decide what's right for you. My own information on MyLifeLine.org is public, so feel free to check it out if you want by searching on my name.

After I spent some time thinking about what I needed, I sent the following e-mail to a wide audience:

Dear Friends and Family,
I am always learning to ask for what I need, and getting better at it all the time. Neither my needs nor my problems have changed one iota, really, during this experience. They are only magnified by it. Everything seems harder (laundry, errands, groceries, work, etc.) or more pronounced (loneliness, fear, and anxiety) or takes longer (writing thank you notes, walking, and returning phone calls). You can help if you are next door or 7,000 miles away. Here's how: Sign up to receive my updates online. Repeating the same story multiple times is just not an option. I don't have the energy. If you see friends or family who should be on the list, and aren't, please share the information with them.

(*continued*)

(*continued*)

What I Need:

1. Invite me to do stuff with you—picnics, concerts, movies, parties, meals, walks, happy hour, etc. It is sometimes tough to plan things because I never know how I will feel, so feel free to also just call spur of the moment and say, "Let's go now." Keep asking me even if I am not feeling up to it the first time.

2. Call to check on me periodically or drop an e-mail to just let me know you are thinking of me. I love getting cards, but don't want flowers or gifts unless it's something I specifically asked for or a book or movie. There is no room in my tiny condo. If you really want to buy me something, here are some things I could use—New hammock chair for my deck; my old one disintegrated and I miss relaxing out there with a book—A juicer; every book I read talks about the benefits of juicing, and I have many veggies from the garden I could use—Airline miles or ticket vouchers (thanks Darryl & Kay for your generosity of this front already)—itunes gift cards (Abby sent me one this week and I realized this is perfect; because I don't have a TV, I buy episodes online, and music too).

3. Bring me dinner or take me out for brunch or ice cream or coffee!

4. Easy stuff for me to make or eat is helpful because often nothing sounds good and I don't have the energy to cook. Cut up fruit, instant oatmeal packets, yogurt, soup, or other stuff I can freeze (in individual servings is even better), small servings of salads (quinoa, tuna, broccoli, or other healthy stuff), and single serving beverages.

5. Offer your expertise deciphering medical bills or insurance paperwork.

6. Invite me to scrapbook with you (I am so behind).

7. Call and ask, "Do you need anything this week, today, right now?"

8. Send me funny stuff (laughter helps a lot) by mail, e-mail, carrier pigeon.

(*continued*)

(*continued*)

9. Ask me to take a walk (I am slower these days). It is so hard to get motivated to exercise, but I need to walk since I can't do much other stuff.

10. Loan/give me a good book/movie/CD.

11. Offer your volunteer time, expertise, retreat location, or just a donation to support the work I'm doing for singles with cancer. This is important to me as I realize how hard this is without a built in support system.

12. Pay for a Reiki session, a massage, or a cleaning service.

13. Invite me on a road trip, to stay with you for a few days, or spend the weekend at your cabin. I have been staring at my own four walls for a while now.

14. Give me a hug (even a virtual one is not bad). Hold it longer than usual.

15. Drop by with a DVD and some Cherry Garcia.

16. Help me figure out a good, relaxing three- to five-day get-away for the end of treatment so I have something to look forward to. Cancer is expensive, so it should be somewhat easy on the budget too.

17. Tell me you love me (or like me a lot). So many have already done this—Thanks so much!

18. Offer to go with me to chemo or Dr. appointments.

19. Just offer to hang out—it gets lonely not being able to plan fun stuff as usual.

20. Offer to unload my dishwasher, mop my floor, vacuum, wipe down my microwave, or do a quick tub cleansing. This can even be on the way out to a movie!

21. Keep being the great friend, parent, sister, aunt, cousin, co-worker you have always been, and don't be afraid to ask me anything or tell me you don't know what to say. Just saying something is enough. Thanks for being here for me, and for asking what you can do. I hope this helps.

—*Tracy Maxwell*

Download this letter as a Word doc that you can edit for yourself at IAmTracyMaxwell.com.

The response I got to this request was overwhelmingly positive. Almost all of the items on the list were fulfilled by friends from far and near. People flew to Denver to be with me for EVERY chemo session, staying for several days afterward to take care of me when I was feeling my worst. I received hundreds of cards from friends and even friends of friends. Hats, scarves, wigs, and any number of fun and funny gifts also made their way to my door, including journals, frozen food, movies, gift cards, and lots and lots of books.

Most interesting was the positive response I got to the e-mail itself. People were relieved to have some guidance about what they could do, and so anxious to be able to help in some way. The two biggest responses I got from months of treatment were to my e-mail asking for specific help and my post telling people not to worry about saying the wrong thing. I told them anything they said was better than saying nothing, even if it was simply, "I don't know what to say," or "I'm sorry you're going through this."

It is easy to sit at home feeling sorry for yourself about everything you're going through, and lament the fact that people haven't shown up for you as much as you expected. I definitely had those thoughts from time to time. It is much more powerful to remember that everyone is busy going about their own lives. They have no idea what you are going through. You have to actually share, and ASK for what you need. Taking some time to really think about what would be helpful to you, and asking for it, will pay huge dividends. It is not always easy to know, and your needs will even change over time, but don't overlook this important step in the process. If someone said to you, "I need a hug," would you think he or she was weak? I doubt you would. You would just offer a hug.

Two years ago, I heard about a surf camp for cancer survivors in Maui, and I really wanted to go. Even though the camp, operated by Athletes for Cancer, is free, I couldn't afford the plane ticket. I might never have gone had a friend not suggested that I ask for help in getting myself there. Another friend flies constantly for work, and has more than a million frequent flyer miles. I had asked her before to help support travel scholarships for single survivors to come to my events, but never for help for myself. She happily agreed to secure my ticket with her miles.

People want to contribute to us, and by not asking, we deny them that opportunity. What do you really need right now? Find a way to ask for it and then receive it gratefully.

Are you comfortable asking for help?

If not, what could you do to change that?

Are you a good receiver? How do you know? Examples?

Learning to Receive

Be thankful for the least gift,
so shalt thou be meant to receive greater.
—THOMAS à KEMPIS

What if you gave someone a gift, and they neglected to thank you for
it—would you be likely to give them another? Life is the same way. In
order to attract more of the blessings that life has to offer, you must truly
appreciate what you already have.
—RALPH MARSTON

For some of us, receiving is difficult. It's something I haven't done well in the past. From compliments to help to money, I tended to deflect more than accept. But in order to give, someone also has to receive. This is a cycle that speeds up the more we practice it. Give without receiving and you deny others the opportunity to contribute to you, which in turn makes it more difficult for them to receive from others.

Try This

Some Things to Practice in Order to Learn to Receive

1. Keep a receiving journal to record all the things you receive each day. (Bonus points for things you actually ask for. Even if others don't always say yes, asking is so powerful. Keep doing it.)

2. Practice gratitude for all that you have. (I posted "gratitudes" as my Facebook status for several weeks to do this publicly.) Keeping a gratitude journal is great as well. Write down what you are grateful for every day—at least five things, but as many as you can. Pay attention to repeats. It is OK to be grateful for the same things repeatedly, but be conscious about looking for new things all the time. Be open to the abundance in your life! (Sara Ban Breathnach first popularized the gratitude journal in her book *Simple Abundance*.)

3. Mike Dooley of TUT.com suggests visualizing what you desire in your life without worrying about "how" you might receive it—knowing that thoughts become things.

4. Consciously ask for help at least twice a day whenever possible.

5. Break patterns, doing things that you haven't done or said before—this brings new energy and connections.
6. Check out The Receiving Project and sign up for the free 32-day e-course on the Law of Attraction.

Paying It Forward

Alice, a 31-year-old breast cancer survivor, talked about how much she received from others, including financial support from her parents and even from her church. In addition to a large cash gift to help her pay her property taxes, church members also donated household items she could sell at garage sales. "I could never pay it all back," she said, "so instead I pay it forward."

That is one of my purposes in writing this book: to pay forward all the great advice, share the resources, and offer the hope and inspiration to others that so many have given me. I got a great lesson in paying it forward a month after finishing chemo. I decided at the last minute to fly home to surprise my family for Thanksgiving. I made the decision after finding out they would be hosting a 90th birthday party for my grandfather, who had been diagnosed with pancreatic cancer and given two to six months to live 16 years earlier. I didn't want to miss that!

In my rush to work out all the details of this trip, including borrowing a car at the other end so I could get from the airport to my parents' house two hours away, I left the house without my wallet. At first, I didn't think I would even be able to get on a plane without an ID, but, it turns out, you can. You just have to go through every single security screening, including being patted down and having your luggage hand-searched.

That hurdle cleared, I began thinking about the fact that I had no money or credit cards and a layover on a holiday. Yikes. What if something happened with my flights and I got stuck somewhere? I quickly called a friend and asked him to wire me $80. While I was waiting for the money to come through, I heard an announcement that my flight was delayed. Yikes again. If I missed my connection, I would for sure miss Thanksgiving dinner with my family and stood a better chance of getting stranded somewhere. I headed to my gate and explained to the agent what was happening with me. Was there a direct flight I could get on instead? Turns out, yes, but I would have to hurry. I wasn't sure my cash would be there yet, and shared my concern. She handed me my new ticket and told me to run.

When I turned around, the woman behind me in line, who had overheard my entire story, was holding a $20 bill toward me. Tears sprang to my eyes as I asked for her address to return the money. She told me to pay it forward instead. I got home that day with $100 in cash (my $80 came through too) and spent a fantastic holiday with my family.

Five years later, I also had the opportunity to pay it forward. I had landed in Denver, home from a conference, and was waiting for delayed luggage and a friend who was picking me up. Sitting in the baggage claim area, I overheard a woman talking on the phone. When she hung up, she turned to me and said, "I left my wallet on the plane. How stupid is that?" She was clearly flustered, and started explaining what that would mean for her day. I gathered that her husband was coming to get her from Aspen, but that it would be several hours. She told me they did find her wallet, so she would get it back, but she didn't have any money right now.

I offered her some fruit I had in my purse, and then it occurred to me that this was my opportunity to pay it forward. I told her I was going to find an ATM to get her some money and she said, "If you could just buy me a bottle of water, that would be great. I'll be fine as long as I can take my medicine." She had recently had a root canal and was on prescription pain killers.

When I came back and handed her a $20 bill, she said, "Oh no, I can't take that. Five dollars would be more than enough." When I asked how she planned to eat while she was waiting several hours for her husband, she reluctantly agreed to take the money, but I could tell it was very hard for her to do so. She remarked, "It's so easy to give, and so hard to receive." I shared my own efforts to become a better receiver and my story of someone helping me similarly almost exactly five years earlier.

With tears in her eyes, she thanked me over and over again, and by then I had teared up as well. She had mentioned paying me back several times, and I flatly told her I wouldn't take any money from her, but that she could definitely pay it forward as I had. I told her, "You have given me a great opportunity to pay forward a five-year old favor, and I appreciate your allowing me to do so." She got up and gave me a hug, sat down, and then got up to hug me again.

Have you had opportunities to pay it forward in your life?

What is the nicest thing ever done for you by a stranger?

What things have you allowed yourself to ask for help with? What else could you ask for?

Every Friend Matters

> *Friendship marks a life even more deeply than love.*
> —ELIE WIESEL

> *True friendship is like sound health; the value of it is seldom known until it be lost.*
> —CHARLES CALEB COLTON

> *Your job won't take care of you when you're sick. Your friends will. Keep in touch.*
> —ANONYMOUS

I am lucky to have many good friends who contribute to my life in a variety of different ways. I see some more than others, and though a few drift away, I am constantly making new connections. Each friendship is valuable to me.

Like any relationship, friendships take effort to build and maintain. Some are very casual or are based on more superficial connections like shared hobbies or mutual friends. Others are deeper and more meaningful, built with people you feel you can share anything with. Friendships can grow and fade or die. Sometimes the parting is intentional or painful, and other times it's gradual, the slow weakening of a bond that was once important, and then. . .no longer is.

As the Tracy Lawrence song suggests, when the chips are down, you find out who your friends are. I was lucky enough to have people come out of the woodwork for me when I was diagnosed. Friends of my parents, friends of my friends, and long-lost friends that I hadn't heard from in years found some way to show up for me. Some made donations to the Ovarian Cancer Research Fund in my honor, others sent cards, a few brought food, and every once in a while, someone would make a gesture that would bring tears to my eyes for its unexpectedness or kindness.

Like when my friend Heidi surprised me by renting a bright red Mustang convertible to take me to a series of dreaded doctor's appointments and consultations during a particularly difficult time. Her support, and the wind in my hair, cheered me up immensely.

Or when I returned home after a week away to find my friends had cleaned my entire condo, painted my kitchen, hung curtains and a shelf in my bedroom, built a new bookcase, organized and stocked my pantry, planted wheat grass in decorative pots, bought me a new welcome mat for the front door, and even hung a new piece of art above my fireplace. A pumpkin sat on my kitchen table with a note that read, "We love you and you are NEVER alone." It was signed by half a dozen of my friends who had spent their weekend making my home feel cozier. I was so touched and overwhelmed by their generosity and kindness. Their gift is among the nicest things anyone has ever done for me, and it came at exactly the right time.

Or when my friend Judy prepared a picnic dinner in the park featuring a variety of healthy dishes to support my new diet. Knowing she was there to be my advocate and support me has made all the difference in the world.

I already knew I had great friends, but my experience with cancer reminded me of just how great they were, and how very much I was loved. During my most recent recurrence, friends and family donated $25,000 through a fund-raising campaign to help pay for my alternative treatment that wasn't covered by health insurance.

I recognize how fortunate I was, and also know that I would not have received a fraction of the help I did if I hadn't been willing to share what was going on and ask for it. Alli felt the same way when she was diagnosed with stage IV ovarian cancer and given just a few months to live. Though the prognosis wasn't great, her friends were.

"It was difficult in the beginning," she said, "because I didn't really know what I needed, so my friends just assumed, and sometimes the result wasn't helpful." When pressed for an example, she shared the day a big group of people showed up to clean her condo right after she'd gotten home from surgery. It was a bit overwhelming, but even worse was that her fridge got completely cleaned out, down to condiments being thrown away, and she was in no condition to replace those things.

"At first, I felt guilty about asking for help," she said. "But there was one incident that provided a turning point. I ran out of toilet paper. Someone was coming to bring food that night, and I called to see if she could pick up TP on the way. She was so relieved to have a request, and that was when I realized how important it was to share what I needed."

After that, it was easier to let people help with laundry, groceries, and prescriptions. Those little things made a huge difference, she said, and led to bigger things. People from her church provided meals twice a week for a year, and one friend even went clothes shopping for her. "She would go to the mall for me and bring me options to choose from because I was just too weak to walk around that much."

"I was really lucky," Alli said. "When I was extremely sick and thought I was dying soon, friends made a schedule to be at my house almost every day. They didn't want me to be alone. Another group of people got together and decided I needed distraction and entertainment. We had girls' night regularly that involved movie outings or rentals and they even brought snacks so I didn't have to do anything. That really helped my spirits."

Friends drove her to appointments when she began having seizures and couldn't maintain a driver's license, helped her with flights to participate in camps and programs across the country, helped clean her house, or paid for a service.

Alice said her neighbor fed her dinner every day for a year. "It was a huge deal," she said. "It was often the only human interaction I would have all day."

Other survivors and caregivers I interviewed mentioned how painful it was when friends fell away during cancer treatment.

Aileen said, "I lost so many friends during cancer. Not only did some people not show up for me, they didn't even return my calls." Her boyfriend stuck with her through treatment, but the experience took too much of a toll on their relationship, and two months after she finished treatment they split up. She understands how difficult it was for him. "Co-survivors are going through a lot too," she said, noting that he had already been through this before when his ex-wife's mom died of breast cancer. She said she's still afraid to connect with people because she worries if she gets sick again, they will leave her. But she's trying to look more at what is there rather than focusing on what isn't. "We have to appreciate what we have," she said.

Lila witnessed something similar when she served as caregiver to her friend who died of ovarian cancer. Jo Ellen was in her 50s when she was diagnosed, and she and Lila had been friends for 15 years, mostly as travel buddies. "The most painful thing for me was to know that there were people who disappeared from her life," she said. "It was difficult and surprising to her as well. She got it from a cognitive perspective, but it didn't make it easier for her to deal with." Lila said she was the only one her friend could talk to about things, and emphasized that as a friend, family member, or caregiver, it's important to be upfront about what you can and can't do.

"She had a closer friend who helped with physical care-taking. I was clear that I could lend emotional support and that she could call me anytime, day or night," Lila said. "At some point, I would always ask her, 'How is your soul?' That was my role with her."

The people who come through for you might not be the ones you expect. Lesley, a 36-year-old breast cancer survivor, said, "One of the biggest things I learned was that it's often the people you least expect who show up, and the people you think will be there who disappear when things get rough."

Don't spend a lot of time worrying about who is helping or who is MIA. Just be thankful that someone is there. I felt the same as Lesley, and was often amazed that the people closest to me were not necessarily the ones to help out the most in a crisis, and it is sometimes surprising who does show up when I least expect it. I have learned that things rarely unfold the way I think they will, and not to get bent out of shape that so-and-so has been absent.

I really don't take it personally because we all have busy lives and can't always show up the way we would like to all the time. It doesn't mean anything about me at all, and reading into it that someone doesn't care is unfair to them and painful to me. Perhaps it is more difficult for those closest to us to handle what we are going through, making them more likely to check out. Like Aileen, I would rather focus on who does show up and be grateful for that.

I still struggle with which friends fall into the category of those you can ask to drive you to the airport, or list as an emergency contact, and I think a great deal about the relationships in my life and the place they hold. I try not to get too bothered anymore when friendships fade. People grow apart for valid reasons: our interests, schedules, or responsibilities change. Or we find that we have different needs and seek out new friends to better meet them. I do my best to appreciate the friends that are part of my life at any given moment. There are many. You know who you are.

Who are the friends in your life you can count on when the chips are down?

Which friends have you helped and supported?

With whom would you like to cultivate a closer friendship?

2

You Have Options

*The way a team plays as a whole determines its success. You
may have the greatest bunch of individual stars in the world, but if
they don't play together,
the club won't be worth a dime.*
—BABE RUTH

*Fit no stereotypes. Don't chase the latest fads.
The situation dictates which approach
best accomplishes the team's mission.*
—COLIN POWELL

The entire cancer experience is often completely overwhelming. For many
patients, there is also a time crunch for making decisions and starting treatments that can add to the pressure. It is important to know that you have
many options for how you handle things, and that you can always choose
the ones that are best for you. You will receive lots of advice, and hear many
stories of how other people navigated this experience, but your experience is
yours alone, and you get to decide what works best for you.

There are a ton of treatment options, books, programs, scientific studies, seminars, blogs, articles, support groups, and people with opinions. Take a deep breath, prepare yourself to listen to your own inner guidance, and make the choice that is right for you. No matter what anyone else has to say on the topic, including your doctors, you are in charge.

As a single person, it may not seem as if you are part of a team, but you are. Your team involves your health care providers and your support network, and your course of treatment is the game plan. Lots of people will have opinions about how you should proceed, especially your family, your friends, and your doctors. Without a partner to help you make decisions, all of this advice from other quarters could seem overwhelming. Listen to the advice and guidance, but make decisions that are right for you and fit with your beliefs and values.

Step 1: Choose How You Want to Be

How you want to proceed on this journey begins with how you choose to be about it. Often we jump right into doing something, especially in a crisis situation, but how you are being will impact everything else, so it is important to think about that first. It may not seem as if you have any control over how you are going to be through cancer, but you absolutely do. Are you going to be calm and measured, frantic and scared, upbeat and positive, terrified and hasty? Peaceful? Open? Relaxed?

You may well be all of the above at different times, but you can be intentional about how you are going to be as you navigate the process. Some people choose to be passive, allowing the experts to make decisions about what treatment is best, others do their own research, read everything in sight, and are more involved in deciding the best course of action. Whatever you choose is fine, but be intentional about choosing.

How you are being about cancer, optimistic or defeated, will definitely impact your experience, so make a choice from the get go. You will stray from time to time no matter what, but you can always pull yourself back to how you want to be. There will always be people who will suggest you should be another way—more aggressive, more serious, less anxious, more optimistic, and so on, but you get to choose what is right for you. You have many, many options to choose from, and how you decide to be may change throughout your experience as well. This simple concept can drastically impact your journey.

Try This

Who Are You Going to Be?

Take out your journal or a piece of paper and write down everything you are feeling as a list rather than a narrative. Example: scared, unsure, overwhelmed, panicked, alone, frustrated, nervous, and so on. After you have made an exhaustive list, close your eyes and just sit with those feelings for a few minutes. Open your eyes and make another list of your ideal states of being. Take as much time as you need to come up with a really good list. Example: supported, peaceful, blessed, safe, open, joyful, free, loved, and whatever other states of being come to mind for you. Then, from your list, choose how you are going to be right now. You can choose a state of being for an hour, a day, a week, or a month. Whenever you are feeling something other than your ideal, ask, "What would it look like if I were being peaceful (or whatever you choose) right now?" This will give you an action to take to fulfill your ideal way of being in the face of your illness. Whenever you feel the need, choose a new way of being, as often as you like.

Step 2: Choose Your Medical Team

With a serious illness, specialists are often referred by the diagnosing physician or dictated by those who fall within your insurance network. Because patients are overwhelmed with the implications of their new diagnosis, it is easy to just accept the doctor you've been "assigned," but choosing a health care team is one of the most important decisions you will make. These professionals could be a part of your life for years to come. It's not impossible to change providers if you're not happy, but it's far better to choose wisely from the beginning, and take the time required to find the best fit for you. Kris Carr called herself the CEO of Save My Ass Technologies in her documentary *Crazy, Sexy Cancer,* and interviewed several doctors to find the right one for her. Though she was in New York City, she chose a doctor in Boston. I live in Colorado, but got two second opinions at MD Anderson Cancer Center in Houston. Don't limit yourself.

Give some thought to what is most important to you. What do you like about your current doctors? What bothers you about them? It is perfectly acceptable to ask for the names and contact information for current or former patients to call as references. There are also online sites that provide doctor ratings and information, but my advice is to use those sparingly, giving more weight to actual patients you can talk with. It's even better if they have a similar diagnosis to yours or are similar in age or other factors.

To help make your decision, I suggest bringing a friend or recording your initial meeting with a new doctor (few doctors will mind if you want a digital record of the meeting, but be sure to ask their permission.) This way, you'll have the benefit of a trusted second-opinion or the ability to go back and listen to your conversation again later. Did the doctor answer your questions fully? Did he or she seem distracted or rushed? Were there a lot of interruptions? Did he or she seem concerned with your emotional well-being in addition to your physical health? These are all factors to consider when choosing a doctor.

Questions to ask when choosing a doctor:

1. How many cases of my particular disease have you dealt with?
2. What were the results in those cases?
3. What is the latest research on my disease?
4. Who else might you be consulting about my case?
5. Is there a cure for my disease? If so, what is the cure rate? What is the most likely scenario?
6. How much emphasis do you put on the role of diet, exercise, and stress-management or well-being in general?
7. What complementary therapies do you recommend?
8. What do you think about integrative medicine in general?
9. What is your overall philosophy about health and wellness, cures, and healing?
10. How available are you if I have questions? With whom in the office will I be able to speak? Will you share your e-mail address or cell phone number?

Once you have chosen your team, it is crucial to ensure that they are talking with each other. If your team isn't communicating well, it can make it more difficult on you, and you already have enough to worry about. I ran into challenges when my oncologist's office wasn't providing up-to-date information to my naturopath, and also when I received contradictory advice from my surgeon and oncologist.

One of them suggested one test, the other a different one. I had my own feelings about which tests I wanted to do, favoring those that emitted the least amount of radiation first (I was shocked at how much radiation there is from CT scans) and those that were less invasive or expensive. My insurance company also covered a bigger percentage of some tests than others. These were all factors in deciding which tests and scans to do. I am glad that at one point a technician reminded me that it's my life and I get to decide or say no at any point. Make sure each of your health care providers has the contact information for your entire medical team and knows that all scans and tests should be sent to everyone on that list. Ask to be cc'd on all e-mails and correspondence so you know what's happening, and what isn't.

What qualities are most important to you in a health care provider?

What will make you feel the most comfortable and confident that you are receiving the best possible advice and care?

What are deal-breakers for a health professional?

Step 3: Choosing What You Are Going to Do

This step depends upon your diagnosis, your lifestyle, your health insurance coverage, and a number of other factors. There are myriad options for treating cancer these days, or you may decide not to treat it at all. Many people have made this choice when the treatment would affect quality of life, the time remaining seemed limited, or for a variety of other reasons. Some have made the choice to enjoy the time they had left rather than spend it hooked up to IVs. In some cases, the cancer has even disappeared when patients quit their jobs, released their stress, and began enjoying their lives more.

Most of the people I interviewed for this book took part in conventional cancer treatments, and many were satisfied with the results, at least for a time. Some dealt with severe short- and long-term side effects. Others, like me, had recurrences. A few have had secondary cancers as a result of their original treatment. There is no guarantee with any course of action. Each person has to choose what he or she is most comfortable with.

Brian said of his treatment, including a stem cell transplant and high dose chemo, "It was barbaric. It's horrendous to go through that. I'm traumatized from the treatment."

A 2010 participant in a canoe trip I organized for single survivors was originally diagnosed with cancer as a teenager and has since had two recurrences as a result of the treatment she received years ago. In her late 40s, she's still experiencing effects from her childhood cancer. Another friend later had a stroke in his 30s as a result of treatment for his brain tumor in college. When we are diagnosed and operating from fear, we rarely take the time to understand the long-term implications of our current treatment decisions, but we should.

Several other single survivors I spoke with mentioned post-traumatic stress disorder (PTSD) or other trauma from their treatment experience. Alice said, "I thought this would be a six-month issue. I had no idea that three and a half years later, I would still be too sick to work from menopause and other problems, and dealing with clinical depression and PTSD."

Personally, I wish I had known more about alternative treatments from the beginning. I found this path later, and mostly on my own, as I didn't know anyone personally who had chosen this route. I read books and did my own Internet searches to learn more about it, and eventually found a number of CAM (complementary and alternative medicine) practitioners that I felt comfortable with, including naturopaths, Chinese medicine doctors, acupuncturists, herbalists, chiropractors, Reiki masters and massage therapists, and energy healers, as well as alternative clinics and nutritional detox programs.

Heather Swift, now a nurse, said she would have made different choices as well. "I might not have done chemo. I would have followed more holistic therapies," she said. "I would have managed side effects with acupuncture and different practices." She continues, "In some ways we can do more harm than good with practices that are unnecessary. I have late effects from the treatment—chemo brain still years later, cognitive difficulties, bouts of depression, neuropathy in my hands and feet, sexual side-effects including decreased libido, early menopause, and fatigue."

Treatment options are varied, but you will likely only hear about the "standard of care" from your medical team. They are required by law to prescribe this tried and true path for each different type of cancer because it is the one that is most accepted. Do some research on your own before making decisions about your primary treatment, as well as complementary therapies that can help with side effects. I will share some limited information about various therapies here, but there are too many to list them all. A healthy diet is key no matter what approach you take, but MDs receive very little nutritional training in medical school, so you aren't likely to hear much about this from most doctors.

Integrative or Holistic Medicine

This approach is not meant to cure disease. Rather, it provides support to overall health by focusing on the whole person, which makes it easier for the body to heal, and provides relief to common cancer complaints. This approach is not either-or, and is often called complementary, as it is often used in conjunction with more conventional therapies.

While often called "nontraditional" modalities by practitioners, many of the therapies used are actually much older and more well-established than modern medicine. Examples include: acupuncture, Reiki, or other energy healing; massage, chiropractic, and body work; herbal and other supplements as well as various smoothies and juicing; and biofeedback, yoga, meditation, and other stress-reduction techniques.

There is a tremendous amount of science behind the efficacy of these approaches as well, and more and more hospitals and clinics are developing some type of Integrative Medicine departments, classes, or support. Additionally, numerous alternative medicine clinics are operating around the world with tremendous success. Doctors such as Andrew Weil, Dean Ornish, Bernie Siegel, and Lissa Rankin have lent significant credibility to this growing field.

Diet

You have so many options about what to put into your body as fuel. Why not choose the healthiest ones? Especially now, your body needs to be in peak condition. Like many others, I believe food is medicine. Now is the perfect opportunity to consider your food options and make better choices.

I was drawn to a healthier way of life before cancer forced my hand, but don't think I ever would have pursued it without a significant motivation. Now I choose to eat a healthy, whole food, mostly vegan diet. I largely gave up sugar, white flour, meat, dairy, and most processed foods. There are certainly many examples of people who have cured their disease with diet alone, but I use a more balanced approach. I explain my new way of eating this way: food is not necessarily going to cure my cancer. The body is a wonderful mechanism and can digest anything we feed it, but some things are more difficult to digest than others, so if the body is working harder to digest the food I eat, it doesn't have as much energy or focus for immune function. There are foods that boost the immune system and reduce inflammation, and those are beneficial when dealing with disease, so I would rather eat those foods whenever possible.

Want to know the biggest surprise of all? It was way easier than I anticipated to eat this way. For four years between my first diagnosis and subsequent recurrence, I became aware of the tremendous health benefits of this type of lifestyle, but I wrote it off as impractical. I decided I couldn't do it before I even tried. Now that I'm actually doing it, I can report two things for sure: 1. It does take some adjustment and time to figure out how to live this way and 2. It is absolutely possible for anyone to do it.

The big-time upside is that I look and feel great. My skin is amazing, I've lost 40 pounds, I have more energy, and my fingernails are three times stronger. Though it wasn't the goal, I went from a size 12 to a size 6 in about 14 months. The best part is that I feel better than I have in my life! I have so much energy, and none of the minor aches and pains, stomach issues, or gas that used to be prevalent.

I was so worried about all the things I would have to "give up" in order to be healthy. Dairy? Really, is it that bad for you? After reading *The China Study*, I now have no doubt. No more ice cream or cheese? I have found great dairy-free ice cream alternatives (made with coconut and almond milk and natural sweeteners), and haven't missed cheese nearly as much as I thought I would, though when I do cheat, just a small serving is satisfying. I also choose healthier options such as goat cheese and coconut milk yogurt. I have been really shocked that I don't seem to crave previous favorites very often. My palate has definitely changed.

I do admit to falling off the wagon occasionally, usually when faced with some type of comfort food that brings back fond memories or when I am starving and nothing healthy is available. I sometimes even crave meat and assume that I need some type of nutrient contained therein. When I do cave and have the chicken wings, pizza, or a cheeseburger, I don't beat myself up, and I realize that these falls can actually be beneficial as I remember how terrible I feel afterward. This is part of finding a balance. If you eat healthy all the time and are resentful and angry about "having" to make that choice, the stress involved counteracts any benefits you are getting from the diet. Again, it is important to make choices that work for you and not beat yourself up about them, whatever you choose.

Make Changes Slowly

You don't need to change your entire diet all at once. One of my favorite approaches comes from *The Engine 2 Diet* by Rip Esselstyn. This book details how a firehouse in Texas began eating a mostly vegan diet by eliminating items individually over the course of a month—one week, meat, the next, dairy, then sugar, and so on. Mostly, people feel so good at the end of a month that they don't want to go back, but some add back in some foods or categories and do the plan 50 or 75 percent. It's your call, and it's still likely healthier than before.

Freeze Food Ahead or Share

As a single person, it is sometimes difficult to think about planning and cooking a meal just for one person. This was often the case for me, and it was easier to just nuke something single-serving from the freezer. Now I often make a big pot of soup with lots of veggies and freeze it in glass jars (be sure to leave room at the top for expansion or you will find broken glass instead of your next meal.) Get four friends together and make a meal with four freezable servings and trade. You have nearly a week's worth of meals! Or trade cooking with each other once a week so every month you can go to someone else's house for dinner. Food and fellowship all in one!

Start Reading Labels

They list the most prevalent ingredients first, so if sugar, fructose, or the many other names used are listed in the first two to three ingredients, or anywhere, I steer clear of it. I like Michael Pollan's (*In Defense of Food*) recommendation to not eat anything with more than five ingredients or anything you can't pronounce.

Plan Your Meals and Make a Shopping List

Plan a week's worth of meals, and shop for just what you need rather than tossing a bunch of stuff in the cart and figuring it out later. I have stopped throwing lots of food away after it spoiled from sitting in the fridge too long as a result of this practice alone. I share a great shopping list/meal planning tool on my website at IAmTracyMaxwell.com.

Keep Meals Simple

I have never been a great cook, so the simplicity of a whole foods diet really appeals to me. I don't make complicated sauces and numerous dishes—just a mix of good fresh veggies either cooked or raw or simple dishes with three to five ingredients. Steaming takes just minutes, and my meals are generally ready much sooner without so many elements to time just right so everything is done at once.

Put Together a Great Binder Full of Yummy Healthy Recipes

I've filled my binder with recipes from magazines and websites. WholeFoodsMarket.com is a great resource for recipes, buying/storing tips, and inspiration.

Join a CSA (Community Supported Agriculture)

These programs are popping up all over. Buy a "share" in the spring to support the purchase of seeds and the labor of planting crops, possibly donate a little of your own sweat equity in weeding and watering, and reap the benefits of a big box of fresh produce every week through the summer and fall. I go in with friends though, as the shares can yield large quantities of veggies.

Shop at Farmers' Markets

Buying directly from the source has several benefits—you know where your food is coming from and you can ask questions about how it was grown; you eliminate the middle-man, which can save money; and it means your food wasn't packaged and shipped for days to reach you. In addition, you are supporting the local economy and farmers with sustainable practices while creating a smaller carbon footprint at the same time. Win-win-win.

Lifestyle

There are many lifestyle options that can also help you, physically and emotionally. It is important to choose options that best fit your interests as this will encourage you to stick with your regimen. I have listed only a small number here, but there are many more than can help reduce stress and foster well-being.

Balance

Achieving balance in daily life is not easy. Our busy lives force us to live by the calendar and schedule nearly every moment. Some people find success in scheduling time for themselves and honoring it as they would an appointment with someone else. Others do a better job of being spontane-ous in taking time out to rest and relax. Find a way to make time for yourself, whether it is on a daily basis or by working hard for a few weeks at a stretch and then taking an afternoon off. We all need downtime to rejuvenate, and if we don't take it, stress can increase while productivity decreases. Have you ever thought of illness as your body's way of telling you to slow down? Taking time for yourself as often as possible can help to ensure good health.

Once again, finding a lifestyle that works for *you* is key. People have found success with a number of different approaches, and it is OK to experi-ment with what others share, but you may create a way that has never been used before. As long as it works for you, that is what matters.

Yoga

This popular exercise embodies mental, physical, and spiritual disciplines. Created in ancient India as a Hindu practice, modern yoga offers a number of varieties, from power to restorative and everything in-between. Yoga has been shown to provide a number of benefits, from reduced stress to increased flexibility. It can improve mood and decrease anxiety as well as lessen the symptoms of asthma.

Several studies have shown the benefits of yoga to cancer patients in improving sleep, reducing inflammation, and decreasing pain, depression, and fatigue. The hardest part is just showing up on your mat. Once you are there, the rest can be easy, as yoga offers a number of resting poses to allow for a break if the practice becomes too challenging.

Meditation

I used to put so much significance onto meditation, feeling like I had to do it "right," sit in a certain position, have incredible insights each time or work something out. Attending a yoga and meditation retreat and reading Pema Chodron have cured me of those limiting ideas. There is nowhere to get, and nothing to achieve. Meditation, like yoga, is about practice, about showing up. Chodron is an American Buddhist nun, and her straightforward and accessi-ble language is one of the reasons I like her books so much. She has practiced meditation for years, and still suffers from monkey-mind. Reading that helped me realize that meditation is not necessarily something we improve at. Rather, it is just noticing the breath and, when the mind wanders, bringing our-selves back to noticing the breath again. That's it. We are the ones who place so much expectation on a transcendent experience every time. Yes, we may have those kinds of aha moments and magical experiences during meditation, but that is not the goal, and we can't meditate for that purpose. Just showing up and practicing regularly is all that's required. I had trouble even with that until someone said to me, "It doesn't matter what position your body is in—meditate lying down if you have to, before going to sleep or when you wake up." That advice did the trick for me, and now I meditate for 20 to 30 minutes nearly every morning. I don't move at all, and this allows me to meditate even if I'm sharing a room with someone else, without interruption.

Alternative Therapies

Chiropractic   In layman's terms, the spine is the communication mechanism between your brain and the rest of your body. When it gets out of alignment, the bones can pinch the nerves, cutting off communication to parts of the body that particular nerve system connects with. These subluxations can cause huge problems in the normal functioning of organ and other body systems. Though I always thought of chiropractic as a great fix when I was in pain, I now understand that there can be underlying problems for months or years before symptoms such as pain or disease occur. I now receive regular adjustments (several times a week) to get and keep my spine in proper alignment. I began seeing a new chiropractor who did x-rays to determine exactly how my spine was out of whack, and he uses kinesiology to test for what needs adjustment during each visit. We do a follow up x-ray after a few months to see what progress has been made and what still needs work, and visits become less frequent.

Acupuncture   One of the oldest healing practices, and one traditionally associated with Chinese medicine, acupuncture involves tapping into the body's energy channels or meridians. Studies have shown that this method can be as effective or more so than drugs for controlling pain and nausea. Chinese medicine suggests that imbalance is the source of illness and is created when the flow of energy or qi is blocked. The proper placement of needles is said to reopen the channels, allowing energy to move freely throughout the body. I was first introduced to acupuncture when it was offered in my oncologist's office by a traditional Chinese medicine (TCM) doctor. The first day I saw him, I was amazed at what he could tell about me from taking my pulse and looking at my tongue for a few minutes. My sister was with me, and her jaw was on the floor as he accurately described my personality before beginning treatment using only those two simple techniques. I have used this treatment since then to control menopause symptoms, including hot flashes, induced by cancer treatments.

Massage   Prior to joining the board of an organization that offered massage for free to cancer patients following treatment, I had never thought of massage as having therapeutic benefits; rather, it was just something I did occasionally when I wanted to treat myself to a spa day. I took advantage of the services of re-org Denver and discovered tremendous relaxation, stress-relief, and pain management benefits. Studies have shown again that it can decrease stress, anxiety, depression, pain, and fatigue. Because massage can impact the lymph system, helping to move toxins out of the body, it is not always recommended for those with certain types of cancer. Do your own research, and ask your doctor before getting a massage during treatment.

Energy Work   Like acupuncture, Reiki also focuses on the energy meridians in the body through a method that involves light touch. I was first introduced to this Japanese healing method when I was going through chemo. A local organization in Denver, called LifeSpark, offers reduced cost Reiki to cancer patients for three months during treatment, and my friends were generous enough to pay for it for me. I also had friends who sent me Reiki long-distance. I was interested enough in this noninvasive practice that now I am learning Reiki and have been attuned to practice it. Almost every night, I practice on myself before going to sleep. It relaxes me, and makes sleep come more easily—something I have sometimes had issues with in the past.

Weighing Your Options

There is so much conflicting information out there these days. I understand how difficult it can be to determine who you can trust, and to decide which approach is best for you. Only you can do that. I did a tremendous amount of reading, talked to other survivors, interviewed practitioners, and listened to my gut to make decisions about my treatment plan, and it changed from time to time. I would see my naturopath for a while and take lots of supplements, and then my system would be in balance and I would take a break. Then I might see an acupuncturist or other energy healer, or get some coaching. I was sporadic at best with juicing, but recognize the benefits of making these practices routine. It is important to be gentle with yourself. Treatment can be like a full-time job whether it is conventional or alternative or a holistic combination of all of the above. You can only do what you can do, and beating yourself up about not doing more just doesn't serve you.

Career and Finances

Single survivors face unique challenges when it comes to working through treatment and maintaining health coverage. Most expressed the dichotomy between needing to work to maintain health insurance and feeling too sick to take care of themselves, much less work, during treatment. Many went on disability or other forms of assistance during treatment. Additionally, many are young adults just beginning careers, with little sick leave and perhaps without health insurance altogether. The new health care law will affect a huge number of patients in this population, and ensure that more are covered, regardless of employment status. This allows for better preventative medicine, and possibly more treatment options in general. The new coverage may even provide for more alternative therapies. There is still much that remains to be seen as the law goes into effect.

A few of the perspectives from solo survivors about this issue:

"Financial issues continue to affect me following treatment. My income was drastically reduced because I wasn't able to sustain the long work hours. I am also concerned about how missing so much work affected my career. I may be perceived as less reliable, my performance and turnaround time on projects were likely affected by absences or being tired or sick."

"I was terminated without cause and with no documented performance issues five days after disclosing I was being treated for breast cancer."

"Financial concerns are the number one problem for me hands down. I am massively in debt with no end in sight. I cannot begin to dig myself out and there is more on the way."

"Medical coverage is a nightmare! I must stay employed full-time to have benefits, but cancer treatment is like a full-time job in and of itself. I have crazy high health insurance costs and co-pays. I feel like I'm drowning."

"I had to travel for treatment, and living expenses in a different city were bank-breaking."

"It would be nice for hospitals and doctors' offices to help patients through the financial and insurance maze."

"I had just started a new job and wasn't eligible for health care yet. One week in, I had a seizure and found out I had a brain tumor. Luckily, COBRA covered me, and my work took pity on me and held my job for four months while I was treated. After being back for two months following brain surgery, I had to leave again, but since I didn't have 90 days in, I didn't qualify for insurance or sick leave or family medical leave, so then I had no income and no way to pay for COBRA. If I was married, I could have been covered under my spouse's plan and that would have been nice."

"Being able to support yourself is another major concern of being single. If I'm too sick to work, what happens? If I lose my insurance, what happens? How do I afford this? There is no one else for me to rely on."

"I am on disability at the moment, but it doesn't cover all the bills by a long shot. I am hoping to work for myself, but not sure how I'll get insurance. Worries about money make everything worse, and it's already hard enough."

"I never got to establish any sort of career, and at this point, I work customer service part-time. I feel really limited to just do that my whole life because my treatments make it pretty impossible to do anything else."

"I couldn't work during treatment, so my boyfriend paid for everything except my health insurance, and my parents paid for that. I also couldn't afford a lot of holistic healing, but lots of people helped me out—comped me or bartered. I was so grateful for their support."

From these comments, it can seem as if options are limited in this area. It is easy to see the problems, and more difficult to recognize solutions. This is another area where your community is crucial if you are willing to reach out. Little can produce more shame than financial struggle, and feeling alone with it can truly compound this stress. Asking for help can make all the difference in the world.

Alice described the financial struggle as humiliating as she went from making $20,000 a month to living on $1,500 from disability and being on food stamps, and eventually losing her house and filing for bankruptcy. "Because of waiting periods for social services, some months I had no income, and the process for filing was complicated and confusing. I was just building my business, so I didn't have savings. I was lucky I had health insurance. It certainly would have been easier with a spouse to support me." She said there were so many big decisions to make about treatment, fertility, and finances that Alice admits she made some poor choices about the latter.

Heather Swift said, "I didn't have health insurance. My ex was working at a coffee house with no insurance. I ended up on Medicaid. I had no concept of what that was or that it even existed before. I STILL have medical bills that I'm paying off years later. I got a job at a bakery and took the bus there at 2:00 a.m. The kids went with me and slept there while I worked. Then I could be with them during the day. I got just a few hours of sleep on a good day. I did everything I could during that time to make any money. If I could pick up a shift during the day and get tips, I did. I bought clothes at garage sales, swapped and bartered for things we needed."

The bottom line is, you do not need to struggle alone. There are resources available to help you. The difficult part of accessing various resources can be overcoming our own pride or any sense of shame we feel that we can't do it ourselves. Of course we can't. That's why these services and programs exist. A social worker at your doctor's office should be able to help you research and pursue options suited to your circumstance. Asking can be the hardest part, and is the most important first step.

Try This

Sources of Financial Support

- Get an appointment with a social worker at your doctor's office or hospital, ask for help in figuring out the finances, and appoint a friend or family member to help manage bills, insurance claims, and other financial issues.

- Apply for financial assistance from as many sources as you can find. There are a variety of programs and services through the government and specifically for cancer patients through private foundations. The LIVESTRONG Foundation is a good starting place for more research on this topic.

- Set up a crowd-sourced fund-raising site to help get funding from a number of sources instead of just one. When friends and family can all give a small amount, you can raise money quickly by spreading out the giving from a number of sources. I used GiveForward to raise money for my alternative treatment, and was very pleased by how easy it was. My friends and family contributed more than $25,000 in a matter of weeks.

- If the cost of an alternative or complementary therapy is preventing you from trying it, there are many nonprofits who offer Reiki, healing touch, massage, yoga, meditation, and other practices free of charge. Do a web search to find programs in your area, or ask providers if they would be willing to provide services at a discount or pro bono. There are organizations such as the Emerald Heart Foundation that provide financial assistance specifically for integrative therapies. Many practitioners in the healing arts will also consider trading services or working out special arrangements. Do you have a friend or relative who would spring for sessions, or can you ask for them as a gift? If a therapy is important to you, find a way to pursue it. Don't rule it out simply because of finances.

- Utilize your disability insurance or medical leave policies to take some time away from work if possible.

- Consider moving in with family or friends during treatment to get help and also save money on rent or mortgage. Having people around all the time also provides a sense of community and may make you feel less alone.

Everyone has to choose the treatment path that works for him or her, and the placebo effect proves that our belief in something has a big impact on whether or not it will work for us. Bruce Lipton's book *The Biology of Belief* helped cement that for me. The best analogy I have is to liken the body to an organic garden. Harsh chemicals are not necessary to create an environment to grow healthy food or have a healthy body. Bugs, pests, and weeds can be dealt with when the environment is balanced, the same way that germs, viruses, and other threats can be dealt with in the body with the right food, exercise, and thoughts that reduce inflammation and boost the immune system.

The most important thing to remember is that you always have options. If one approach isn't working for you, try another, or better yet, utilize a variety of practices to contribute to your overall health and wellness. Rely on your support network to help you research and choose the best options for you. Talk with your doctors, coaches, a therapist, social worker, or medical advocate about what you are dealing with, so they can help you find solutions. There are so many options available. Find the combination that is right for you, and know that it will likely change from time to time.

What practices mentioned in this section appeal to you? What would you need to do to incorporate them into your life?

How well do you manage stress? What actions could you begin taking now that would make a difference?

Step 4: Choose Your Support Network

This is a huge issue for single patients who don't have the built in support from a partner or spouse. There are many sources of support for many different types of needs. You might find yourself needing support for practical matters like getting to doctor appointments or childcare, or for emotional issues such as depression or sadness. You may need help weighing various treatment options or writing a living will. Or perhaps you just want someone to talk to. Do you choose a professional, a family member, a friend, someone who has been through a similar experience, a support group, or a combination of all of the above?

There are so many resources and programs available. Some are listed in the back of this book, but it is definitely not even close to being an exhaustive list. Reach out to one or two to get some guidance, and don't be afraid to change your mind if something isn't a fit. You may join a support group only to find it is adding to your sadness to hear other people's stories rather than helping you. Either find another group, or seek a different path.

Some people choose to be completely open about their illness and seek support from their community like I did, and others, like Krystal, keep it mostly to themselves, telling only a few close friends or family. "It was especially hard for me because I hid that I had cancer," Krystal said. "Only my immediate family and very closest friends knew. You couldn't tell from the outside that I had cancer. I'm just a private person in general, and I didn't know anyone who had had cancer before, so I felt like if everybody knew I would be overwhelmed with sympathy and calls and I just didn't want it. I didn't want the questions and concern."

Wait to Tell

Early on, I got great advice from a friend to wait until I had processed all my own emotions to share my diagnosis. He warned me that I would be deluged once it was public, and that it could be overwhelming. Because I also didn't know any details about my cancer type, stage, or next steps for at least a week, it was great advice to keep it close to the vest for a while until I could share more information.

It is easy to rely on those who show up—parents in some cases, or close friends—but you do have options when it comes to choosing your support team. You made a list of all the communities you belong to and the people in them in chapter 1. If you haven't already reached out to the people on that list, do so now to ask for support. Make a list of what you need help with (see the one that follows as a starting point), and allow people to self-select the ones they can fulfill or ask specific people to take on certain roles. You can even let someone else take on the role of filling these positions for you, by reaching out to others on your behalf.

Carefully consider who will fill the role of your medical advocate. My gynecologist asked me one day who was helping me make my treatment decisions. I told her about all my wonderful friends and my family. She said, "It is great that you have so many people supporting you, but you need *one* person who can help you with this." Her advice: choose one person to be your advocate, to know all the information, to go with you to doctor appointments when possible and to be your sounding board. That is what had been missing for me during my first round of treatment. There was always someone with me at doctor's appointments and hospital visits, but not one consistent person. Choosing one friend to be my medical advocate has made all the difference, and it was much easier than making decisions by committee.

Whether it is researching doctors, managing medical bills and insurance issues, organizing volunteers and meals, or providing emotional support, there are people in your life who have natural abilities and skills in each of the areas in which you need help. Be clear from the beginning about what you need, and be sure they can fulfill the role. If they can't, or aren't, find someone else who can. This will help make sure you have the best person in place for the various tasks you need handled.

Your Support Team (brainstorm some possible team members to help out or have someone else take on this role for you)

- Medical advocate
- Emotional support
- Doctor visits
- Physical needs
- Organizing files
- Communicating with others
- Medical bills and insurance issues
- Transportation
- Meals
- Childcare (if needed)
- Cleaning
- Other

You have so many options. (Tired of hearing that yet? You do though!) You can research these on your own, or ask someone on your team to take this on for you, but if you are open about what is going on with you, people will naturally reach out to tell you what they know. I discovered so many programs and services from Chemo Angels to the LIVESTRONG Summit from friends and even friends of friends. As a single person, I found it much easier to be open about what I was dealing with so I could request and accept support. If you choose to be more private, you will simply need to do more on your own. Either way, the choice is yours to make.

3

You Are Responsible

In the long run, we shape our lives, and we shape ourselves.
The process never ends until we die. And the choices
we make are ultimately our own responsibility.
—*ELEANOR ROOSEVELT*

I am free because I know that I alone am morally
responsible for everything I do.
I am free, no matter what rules surround me. If I find them
tolerable, I tolerate them; if I find them too obnoxious, I break
them. I am free because I know that I alone am morally
responsible for everything I do.
—*ROBERT HEINLEIN*

If you could kick the person in the pants responsible for most of your
trouble, you wouldn't sit for a month.
—*THEODORE ROOSEVELT*

You, and you alone, are responsible for your life. It is tempting to blame others or circumstances or just dumb luck for what happens to us, but it is much more empowering to take responsibility, if not for everything that happens to us, at least for how we respond to it. It is easy to feel like a victim when we get sick. It doesn't feel as if we have control over what is happening to us as we are carried along on the roller-coaster ride of serious illness. But I've found it's much more empowering to take responsibility for who I get to be in this situation and even for my health itself.

Being responsible for my health meant that I followed up with my gynecologist after my ER visit as recommended. It has required me to schedule appointments and scans as needed, and to request information when it hasn't arrived as expected. It means that if I don't have enough information to make a decision about something, it is up to me to get it. It means not blaming others, my work, or circumstances when I don't eat as well as I planned, get enough sleep, or find time to exercise.

Being responsible for your health includes trusting your own instincts, insisting upon more tests when you know something is wrong, being your own advocate when it comes to your treatment and care, choosing what works best for you, and making the time to take care of yourself.

Intuition

All great men are gifted with intuition. They know
without reasoning or analysis, what they need to know.
—ALEXIS CARREL

A woman uses her intelligence to find reasons
to support her intuition.
—GILBERT K. CHESTERTON

It's been described as a still small voice deep inside each of us, a whisper, a gut feeling. A lot of people dismiss intuition as a fantasy or daydream of the conscious mind. I used to. But on my cancer journey, I've realized my intuition is something deeper that can be trusted. Intuition whispers and calms, and invites us to step into a better way, and because it's so soft and nonintrusive, we often miss it or, even worse, hear it and dismiss it.

I dismissed my intuition for so long because I didn't recognize it. This important voice is often obscured by the ego, which is much louder. Our ego tries to protect us from making a fool of ourselves, and is there to protect our often fragile perception of who we are. Intuition exists to bring forth our highest self, which often requires us to take risks that seem threatening to the ego.

At a retreat for cancer survivors at the famous Miraval Spa in Arizona, I attended a program on intuition. At one point we were asked to partner with someone next to us who we didn't know and exchange a personal item—a piece of jewelry or clothing. We were led through a brief meditation to get centered and then told to pay attention to any messages we were getting about the person whose item we held.

Immediately, I saw images of a beautiful brown horse, and almost as instantly, I dismissed them as not the real message I was supposed to be focusing on. My logical brain reasoned that these images were only coming to mind because I knew, of course, that Miraval is famous for its Equine Experience. I had been hearing about how amazing this program was since the minute I'd set foot on the property. I forcefully tried to clear the horse images from my mind so I could sense something personal about this woman sitting next to me. The horse popped up again and again and I got so frustrated. The entire exercise was less than 90 seconds long, but I made myself wrong for most of that time.

When the facilitator asked us to share with our partners, I reluctantly told her what I had seen. She exclaimed, "I JUST finished the Equine Experience and it was one of the most amazing things I've ever done." When I described the horse I had seen, she confirmed that indeed her horse had fit that description. Wow!

She told me in turn that when she held my ring in her hand, she wanted to slump to the floor and take a nap. I shared that I had just come from one of the most relaxing yoga classes I'd ever taken, and had actually fallen asleep at the end of shivasana. I do yoga regularly and that had never happened to me before. They had to wake me up as the next class began filing into the studio.

The stories shared by other participants around the room were equally amazing. They ranged from images, like mine, to physical sensations and even emotions. One woman got a pain in her hand, and her partner confirmed that she had severe arthritis in that exact spot.

This exercise served to show me how easy it is to tap into our intuition and how accessible it is when we choose to listen to it. The more we listen, the more available it is to us. Intuition defies logic, analysis, conventional wisdom, and other tools we often turn to in order to make decisions. Learning to listen for and trust your own intuition will lessen your need to work so hard at figuring it out. Instead, it is possible to just know what is right for you.

There were two times that my intuition actually played a role in saving my life. The first had to do with cancer. I was scheduled for a follow up ultrasound in October and ended up getting it in July instead. My doctor called me late on a Friday afternoon to ask me why I had gotten the test early. I didn't even realize I had. She told me it was a good thing I did, because something had shown up, and I ended up having surgery in September.

The second time was more direct as I woke up with a start in the middle of one cold November night. It was the first cold night that fall in Colorado, and my intuition told me something was wrong with my heater. I immediately turned it off and opened the windows. The repairman told me the next day that I needed a new furnace and there was a good chance the old one was emitting carbon monoxide. I didn't have a detector then, but I do now.

What is your intuition telling you about your life? Your course of treatment? Did intuition play a role in your diagnosis? Over and over again, survivors have told me they "just knew" something was going on long before they had any symptoms or tests turned up any problems. It is important for us to listen when we receive messages from our internal guidance system, even if it doesn't make sense at the time. Listening could make a huge difference in your life, possibly even save it.

Are there times in your life when you ignored an intuitive feeling?

Can you think of a time when you listened to your intuition?

What is the benefit of trusting this higher part of yourself?

Our Uniqueness

What each must seek in his life never was on land or sea.
It is something out of his own unique potentiality
for experience, something that never has been and never
could have been experienced by anyone else.
—JOSEPH CAMPBELL

There is a vitality, a life force, an energy, a quickening, that
is translated through you into action, and because
there is only one of you in all time, this expression is unique.
—MARTHA GRAHAM

We have been told for some time now that genetics largely determines who we become and what diseases we will get, as if the cards were dealt at birth and we have no control over them. The emerging field of epigenetics shows us that is not entirely true. Our behavior plays a large role in which genetic traits actually get expressed. What you eat, how you manage stress, what environmental elements you are exposed to, the quality of your relationships, and how much you exercise and sleep, along with other factors, can all play a role.

This is why I love working with a naturopath, because this modality utilizes a holistic approach which recognizes my uniqueness in determining which supplements in what dosages will actually work best for me. My oncologist recommended I see a naturopath after I completed treatment, but he also expressed concern at one point that the regimen I was following wasn't specifically addressing the cancer. He was right. Naturopaths actually don't claim to cure disease. Their role is to help balance the body's functions for optimal health on the premise that when the body is functioning properly, it is capable of taking care of many problems on its own. Our immune systems are quite powerful when they are optimized.

I was sharing with my naturopath that I was having a difficult time remembering to take a certain supplement regularly. He said something that really got my attention. "If you aren't remembering to take it, your body probably doesn't need it." Wow! I don't think I had ever fully embraced my body's unique ability to know what it needs that completely before. As a mostly vegan, I often eat fish and occasionally meat or eggs when other options aren't available, but also when my body is craving it. I have come to accept that real cravings are our body's way of telling us we need something, and I try to listen to them. We just aren't great at listening these days, often eating for reasons other than hunger. We use food and other substances to fill a void or smother a feeling we don't like.

Did We Inherit Cancer?

Sometimes medical advancements can give us more information than we want to know. With the discovery of the BRCA 1 and 2 genes—mutations of which are responsible for breast and ovarian cancer—women can now find out their risk of developing these two cancers. That is both good and bad news. There are many factors to consider before being tested. Is there a history of either disease in your family? Do you belong to one of the ethnic groups at a higher risk?

The test is expensive, and may or may not be covered by insurance, and there is still a chance of discrimination if you find out you do carry the gene mutation, even though Congress passed an anti-discrimination law to protect against this problem. Perhaps most difficult, though, are the decisions you will face if you find that you are positive. Would you have prophylactic surgeries—removal of your ovaries and breasts—to reduce or eliminate your chances of getting cancer? Many women have. One young woman, Joanna Rudnick, in her early thirties at the time, documented her experience, and others who carried the burden of knowing, in her film, *In the Family*.

Rudnick struggled with her own desire to have children, juxtaposed against the chance that she could die if she waited too long to take preventative measures. In her thirties and single, she heard the ticking of a potential time bomb in addition to the proverbial biological clock.

Someone stated in the documentary that women and men who test positive for this gene mutation feel the same as those of us who are cancer survivors. Many of the same emotional and psychological issues apply. You are forced to acknowledge your mortality, and to make medical decisions that will mutilate your body, but could save your life.

I can understand Joanna's need to do so much research, and talk to other women facing the same decision. Her search allows us to go along for the ride, and will help many women who are also struggling with finding their own path. At one point in the film, Joanna's boyfriend wonders, "Does she only like me because she wants my babies, and she wants them quick?" All single woman of a certain age have probably dealt with this stereotype at some point, and those with a cancer history or probability likely feel it more acutely. As if finding the right person weren't already difficult enough, the added pressure of a deadline just seems so unfair!

Eric inherited the FAP (Familial Adenomatous Polyposis) gene from his mom, and that led to a lifetime of health issues right from birth, as well as numerous cancer diagnoses starting at age 33. While he lives a very full life as a successful businessman, extreme athlete and world-class sailboat racer, he has not been able to keep a relationship since his diagnosis.

"I was dating one woman in the medical profession and she said to me, 'You're fucked.' She knew what my diagnosis meant. We stayed together for a while, and then she left me for her ex-boyfriend because she wanted to have kids. Twelve weeks later she called to tell me she was pregnant with my baby. I didn't think I could have kids, but it turned out to be mine. I told her I would be a father but not a husband because she had hurt me too badly. In the end, she aborted the baby because she was afraid it would carry the same gene that had made me sick."

Talking to him, I had the feeling that Eric has probably lived more than most people in the world, and loved more too, but it has left him jaded that all the women who love him eventually leave for one reason or another. Some want kids, others can't handle what they see as a death sentence. He even dated a fellow cancer survivor for a long time, but one day she told him, "one of the two of us is going to die from this. I have kids to think about. I can't do this." He is still friends with her, and while she has dated many other people, she told him she hasn't found anyone she has cared for as much as him.

> "It bothers me that I'm getting angry as I share these stories again," Eric says. "I hate that the bitterness is there. I have fallen in love so many times, and I have been hurt so many times. I am upset and disappointed in the human race, but at the same time, that's not who I am."

Heredity is somewhat controversial in the cancer world. There are some forms of cancer that are clearly affected by genetics, like those mentioned above where the actual gene has been identified, but others are more ambiguously related, if at all, and our own lifestyle can significantly impact the likelihood of certain gene expressions. In addition to having had ovarian cancer three times, I have also had two minor brushes with skin cancer. A small basal cell carcinoma on my shoulder/back was dealt with in a minor office procedure at my dermatologist's. It's pretty clear that skin cancer is significantly linked to sun exposure, though we do inherit our skin type, so genetics plays a small role as well.

Five stitches later, I will have a small scar, but we got all the margins, so it's all gone this time. I have had two other scary-looking moles removed, but both biopsies were negative. This one was a tiny, innocuous-looking pink bump that I noticed in the spring and didn't really think much about. Meeting a stage IV melanoma survivor in early fall that year lit a fire under me to find a dermatologist when she told me her diagnosis began with a small pink bump on her shoulder in her early twenties.

My chances of getting more of these is higher now, so I will have to be even more vigilant about watching for changes in my skin and using sunscreen. I always figured skin cancer was in my future. I'm fair-skinned, and I life-guarded for eight years starting at 16. I grew up on a lake, I guide whitewater canoe trips, and I live in Colorado—where the elevation puts us closer to the sun's rays and we get more than 300 days of sunshine a year. These are all factors in my likelihood of experiencing more skin cancer, not only my genes.

Emotional Connections to Health

I have always believed physical illness has an emotional connection, and grew up with a dad who almost never got sick. He rarely even got a cold. He was a big proponent of positive thinking, and believed that played a role in his health and well-being. His dad (my grandfather) survived 17 years with pancreatic cancer after being given two to six months to live, and we all believed that his positive attitude contributed to his longevity. I also recognize that while my dad worked really hard, he also took time for himself as often as he could, often fishing or hunting or spending time outdoors. While my body might send me a cold to force me to take it easy with a book, one of my favorite pastimes, my dad managed to do it on his own, so illness wasn't necessary.

In the past, I have been bad about giving myself down time, and often lamented that I "needed a break." Is it possible that played a role in the five broken bones I've experienced over the years? That certainly gave me a break—literally—to recover and rest and have some time to myself. My three bouts with cancer have as well. If I slow down more and take time for myself without guilt, will that mean I stop getting sick? I don't know, but I suspect this plays a role.

Does this mean if you get sick, you have a bad attitude or somehow brought it upon yourself? Absolutely not! This concept goes much deeper than that. Much of the emotional connection to illness is subconscious, and it takes real awareness to come to terms with what might be playing a role for each of us.

I began to understand this better when a seriously stiff neck led a friend to recommend Louise Hay's book *You Can Heal Your Life*. Louise, a cancer survivor herself, provides a list of various emotional issues correlated to common illnesses. Rigidity was associated with neck pain, according to the book. When it asked, "Who is being a pain in your neck?" I knew exactly what the problem was. When I spoke to the "pain in my neck" and apologized for my inflexibility, my pain went away, and it hasn't come back.

I subscribe to Christiane Northrup's belief that we are responsible TO our illness, not FOR our illness. I don't believe we are at fault for being sick. The illness is here, like it or not, but knowing there may be an emotional connection gives me another place to look for solutions beyond just drugs or diet. It means I can take some responsibility rather than feeling powerless to do anything about it. This doesn't mean that I will "fix" my emotions in order to cure my cancer, but perhaps, instead, that my cancer is here to help me see some deeper emotional issues that I can heal for my overall well-being.

I noticed, for example, that I was taking on emotional responsibility for lots of people around me, particularly when they were going through a rough time. This didn't always result in action on my part, but energetically, I was carrying the weight of the world whenever I saw a homeless person or heard about my friends' struggles. I just took them on and worried about them without realizing it. This didn't necessarily serve the other person, but it certainly impacted my health in a negative way. This is just one small example of how our emotions can impact our health. This came up for many of the survivors I interviewed as well. Extreme care-taking of others to the exclusion of your own needs and feelings seems to be a contributing factor for illness.

In *Mind Over Medicine*, Rankin writes about two big questions we can ask ourselves to begin to explore these connections:

1. If your health condition had a message to deliver to you, what would it say?
2. What does your body need in order to heal?

Emily, a 45-year-old cervical cancer survivor, said, "I knew right from the get go that I needed to slow down if I had any hope of getting better." Emily writes a great blog called Holy Sit in which she shares her incredible healing experience that most would label a miracle.

Jeremie, a 46-year-old esophageal cancer survivor, said, "I learned through my cancer experience that sometimes the stuff I worry about is just ridiculous. I catch myself more now and pull back from that. Really, our health is so important, and I try to focus on that now."

In her book *A Return to Love*, Marianne Williamson says that we act always out of either love or fear. When we get sick, we are instantly afraid of so many things including death, not being cared for, being alone, not being able to take care of ourselves, having to rely on others, not being able to have kids, how we will pay for everything, and the list goes on and on. During my most recent recurrence, I have been conscious, perhaps for the first time in dealing with cancer, of not making any decisions from a place of fear. This took an incredible amount of consciousness, but I have managed to do it.

The biggest benefit for me has been in my lack of stress. As my oncologist said to me, "You are realistic about your situation, and not in denial, but you are able to live without worry and fear, and that is such a blessing." My circumstances do not impact my peace of mind in the least. That is not to say that I don't think about cancer, of course I do. I still get concerned when

I have a stomach-ache or experience discomfort. I just don't let that concern consume my life. My worrying about it is not going to make it better, but my belief that I am healing just might, as proven by a growing body of evidence into the mind–body–spirit connection.

Try This
Minimize Distractions

When you are dealing with an illness, the rest of your life doesn't get put on hold. Especially as a single person, managing everything can seem really overwhelming. It is important to minimize things that distract you from taking the best care of yourself that you can. Put volunteer positions on hold, work less if possible, or arrange to work from home a few days a week, and generally limit obligations as much as you can.

Make two columns and list what you can do in one, and what is really making your life difficult in another. Ask for help with those items in the second column. Remember that your friends want to contribute to you, and just need to be reminded about what you need.

Circumstances

Each one has to find his peace from within. And peace to be real must be unaffected by outside circumstances.
—MAHATMA GANDHI

You must take personal responsibility. You cannot change the circumstances, the seasons, or the wind, but you can change yourself. That is something you have charge of.
—JIM ROHN

"We cannot change the cards we are dealt, just how we play the hand," said Randy Pausch, the now-famous college professor and author of *The Last Lecture* who used his terminal pancreatic cancer diagnosis to teach others to really achieve their childhood dreams. While many of us would consider Randy's diagnosis a tragedy, Randy himself focused on living, and his humor and intelligence in the face of death has inspired millions.

I am learning that circumstances don't have to play any role whatsoever in how I feel because I have control over how I perceive my circumstances. It is not so much the circumstances themselves that impact how I feel, but rather the story I tell myself about them. Of course we are going to react immediately to a situation—a job loss, a divorce, a cancer diagnosis, a lottery win—but after the initial shock wears off, we have the opportunity to choose how we frame it. Is it an opportunity or a devastating loss? Is it "good" or "bad?" Most of us see things this way: Win the lottery = good. Get cancer = bad. But these events can precipitate either or both positive and negative outcomes. Many lottery winners end up broke or in debt a few short years after their windfall, and we all know cancer survivors who say their diagnosis was the best thing that ever happened to them (I am one of them). Buddhist philosophy teaches that good and bad things don't happen to us, but rather we put those labels onto the events in our lives and treat them as one or the other.

For a long time, I labeled being single as bad. I told myself I must be single because something was wrong with me, that I was unlovable or unworthy of a lasting relationship. Getting cancer and then having a hysterectomy seemed to confirm it for me; these events were more evidence that I was "damaged goods" and now had even less chance of finding someone who would love me.

The phrase "damaged goods" came up over and over again in my survey of single survivors. One woman described the variety of changes this way: "You are physically changed because of scars, mentally changed because you are damaged goods, socially changed because you don't feel datable, spiritually changed because you wonder, 'why me'?"

I spent years telling myself that life would be so much better if only I could lose 30 pounds. Well, I recently lost nearly 40 pounds because of my healthy diet, and while I feel better than I ever have in my life, going from a size 12 to a size 6 hasn't changed my life perceivably in other ways.

Until recently, I'd thought of the masses in my abdomen as purely harmful tumors to be eradicated. My doctors reinforced this belief, sometimes pressuring me to "do something" about them. An energy healer asked, "What do the masses want from you?" In that moment, both she and I saw them in a new way, as an opportunity to deal with my health differently. Perhaps these masses were here to keep me focused on my health. As I was lamenting to my coach about how tired I was of giving my time, energy, and money to cancer, she responded, "Oh honey, you're not giving all that to cancer, you're giving it to health."

Wow! She is so right. Now I have an entirely different context with which to view these little visitors in my body. What if they are actually here to help me focus on what I am meant to be doing, rather than to harm me in some way? They mostly didn't cause me any problems, and they certainly kept me focused on my health and well-being in a way that I might not have been without them.

Each of these beliefs—that I'm flawed for being single, that my weight determines my happiness, that my tumors are bad—are examples of limiting beliefs, beliefs that limit our ability to live our lives as fully as we are capable of. They can make us miserable if we let them. The way to get rid of these limiting beliefs is to first acknowledge them. Doing so can be tough as these beliefs can be subtle or hidden. Because they're hard to notice, they can unconsciously influence every aspect of our lives for years.

I acknowledged mine by simply paying more attention to my actions and motivations. What did I say to myself when I ate something I "shouldn't"? Found myself for the thousandth time in debt? Got in a fight with my boss? Lost my temper? Misplaced my favorite pair of shoes? As I started listening to myself, I realized how negative and unaffirming I often was. I said things to myself that I would never allow anyone else to say to me.

Once I identified a few limiting beliefs, I worked on letting them go. For some, just being more aware of them helped me to let them go. For others, coaching or EFT (Emotional Freedom Technique) helped. No matter what technique you use, releasing your limiting beliefs can be amazingly transformative.

What have the circumstances in your life taught you?

What do you say to yourself that you wouldn't allow others to say to you?

What limiting beliefs are holding you back?

EFT (Emotional Freedom Technique), commonly called tapping, is a simple self-administered form of therapy. It involves focusing on a specific issue or limiting belief while physically tapping on different parts of your body, the end points of the body's energy meridians.

Practice Letting Go of Limiting Beliefs

Start to listen to what you tell yourself

"I can't."

"I'm broke."

"I'm damaged goods."

"I'm not good at. . ."

Once you uncover the limiting beliefs, there are a number of ways to release them. Seeing them is the first, and often most difficult, part. To us, they aren't limiting beliefs. They are just the way things are. When you recognize that you actually have control over your thoughts, and that your thoughts create your reality, you can more powerfully choose the ones that serve you.

Victimhood

> *If it's never our fault, we can't take responsibility for it. If we can't take responsibility for it, we'll always be its victim.*
> —RICHARD BACH

> *You can be a victim of cancer, or a survivor of cancer. It's a mindset.*
> —DAVE PELZER

My friends and I often joked about when it was appropriate to play "the cancer card." You've probably heard or used this term yourself to describe those times when we pull out our diagnosis as a way to gain favor, sympathy, or some type of advantage. Standing in line with my new friend, Jennifer, at the LIVESTRONG Summit in Austin, she joked that we wouldn't get very far playing the cancer card in this line full of other survivors and caregivers. It's a common joke among survivors—our own version of the "get out of jail free" card. I may have played the cancer card a time or two when going through treatment, and I definitely got some favorable treatment with my bald head occasionally whether I asked for it or not.

As one who believes things happen for a reason, and always looks for that reason, I have said cancer served to teach me to ask for and receive help. There was a distinct moment, though, when I realized how easy it would be to play the victim instead. Going way beyond asking for and graciously receiving the help I needed to get through the experience, I could have used cancer as a way of manipulating others, of getting out of commitments, or of excusing poor behavior. This was a huge aha moment for me as I recognized very clearly the difference between sympathy and pity, and empathy and compassion. There is an instant gratification from victimhood versus the respect and compassion earned through being responsible instead.

No one would question my victimhood if I chose to go that route. I had been through something terrible, faced my own mortality, lost my chance to have children, and suffered the indignities and difficulties of treatment. I had played the victim many times in the past, using whatever status was available to gain sympathy or ask for a break. When I got cancer, though, I saw what playing up all those complaints could get me (mostly more complaints in order to keep the manipulation going), and I made a conscious choice not to do it.

Victimhood isn't always conscious. For some, it's not obvious; it's just the way it is. I'm grateful for the revelation that allowed me to make a conscious choice not to be a victim, and instead to take responsibility for how I respond to the challenge of cancer and any others that life puts in my way, for that matter.

Kelly has dealt with illness for most of her life. Born with a chronic immune disorder, and diagnosed with lupus at 15, she was accustomed to doctor appointments and medications, but getting cancer at 21 added another layer of trauma to what she had already been through. Hospitals, an endless line of specialists, and extreme pain were par for the course for her, but what wasn't part of her routine was talking about her feelings.

"Until a few years ago," Kelly said, "I had emoted approximately three times about my illness. It wasn't allowed. Instead of crying or showing normal emotion, I was a secretive mass of anger and sadness who self-destructed regularly and spoke to no one about how I truly felt."

When she finished cancer treatment she turned to alcohol and pot to dull her pain, and admitted that she did stupid, mean things to her best friend and boyfriend, hurting those who loved her the most. She is still struggling to understand and apologize for her behavior during that time.

"I believed that stoicism equaled strength, and that crying was weakness," she said. "If I divulged the secret devastation of my illness, I wouldn't be the Kelly everyone knew—the one who won class clown in high school."

The anger and depression sunk her, she said, affecting her work, her relationship, and her friendships. Believing no one could understand, she shut out anyone who tried. When her mom forced her into a lupus support group, Kelly sat in the circle with her hands stuffed into her hoody pockets as others, much older than her, shared how hard it was to live with chronic illness.

She couldn't even utilize the comfort of strangers to release her feelings. Instead, she seemed to be on a path of self-destruction, partying and eating crappy food and paying for it with hospital stays. In 2011, after leaving her apartment in New York City to move back in with her parents following a hospitalization, Kelly read about a canoe trip on the Colorado River for single cancer survivors.

Bumping up against her city girl fears of nature—mainly bears, coyotes, and bugs—as well as her disdain for camping, she was also unsure about spending four days with total strangers, but decided to take the risk and flew out to Colorado for three days of paddling and sharing. She bonded with others on the trip, and surprised herself by having fun.

"This trip with fellow cancer survivors literally changed my life," Kelly said. "It opened me up to the possibility of living a full life with illness, without denying its existence. But most of all, it taught me the value of connection, and that changed everything."

No longer the Kelly who dealt with illness in an awful way, used it as an excuse for bad behavior, and hid out from the world, Kelly 2.0—as her fellow trip participants call her—is now training for a 5K, volunteering, learning about her illnesses so she can control them better, and occasionally even eating healthier food.

"I went home from that trip with a sudden interest in playing an active role in my own life," she said.

Solo Survivors

The canoe trip Kelly referenced was sponsored by Solo Survivors, the organization I founded whose mission is to connect single cancer survivors in order that they feel less alone. Offering retreats, adventure trips, support, and coaching. You can find us on Facebook or at SoloSurvivors.com

---

We all face traumas in our lives. They can either tear us down or build us up. How they define us—as a victim or a survivor, for example—is up to us.

Can you identify times that you have played the victim to get support or sympathy?

What does taking responsibility mean to you?

PART

TWO

Survivorship

CHAPTER

4

You Are A Survivor

*Don't be fooled by the calendar.
There are only as many days in the year as you make use of.*
—Charles Richards

*Life is not lost by dying; life is lost minute by minute, day by dragging
day, in all the thousand small uncaring ways.*
—Stephen Vincent Benét

Initially, I was terrified about my illness, and then I was annoyed. I had a life
to live, dammit, and cancer was interrupting it! At the time of my diagnosis,
I was the CEO of a small company, a white-water canoe guide, and an active
volunteer with several different organizations. I had planned to visit Mesa
Verde, spend lots of time on the river, and do some camping that summer.

Just days before Memorial Day, I was told I had ovarian cancer, and
I was instantly ticked that I would have to be recovering from surgery and
starting chemo during the fantastic Colorado summer. I labeled 2006 my
"lost summer" as a result.

Of course, I feel fortunate that I had the luxury of annoyance rather than an overwhelming fear of death. Not everyone is so lucky. Several years and two recurrences later, a friend gave me a beautiful silver bracelet that she had been wearing. I put it on, and then read what it said in small, neat script: Fuck Cancer. I thanked her for the lovely gift, and told her I didn't want it. I just don't see cancer that way.

I'm not suggesting that my experience was fun. I missed out on a lot of things beyond that lost summer, experienced significant dating issues and bouts of low self-esteem, spent a lot of money and time fighting against something that felt at times like an intruder in my body. But I believe "that which doesn't kill you, makes you stronger," and I am still alive. Not only alive, but thriving. Not despite cancer's intrusion into my life but, I believe, because of it.

If it hadn't been for cancer's wake up call, I might still be sleepwalking through life. I might not have ever realized how blessed I am, and how much I have to be thankful for. Cancer does wield some power over me, but it's the power to produce gratitude, to light a fire under me to get going on the things I want to do, and to connect me with other amazing people who have also been forged by this particular fire.

I realize now that instead of interrupting my life, in many ways, cancer has given me a new one. It gave me the courage to leave a job I no longer found fulfilling, to found a nonprofit that focused on hazing prevention, and to find a way to serve other single cancer survivors, including writing this book. It taught me how to ask for help and to really open myself to receiving in a big way. It got me to eat more vegetables and slow down better than anything else in my life ever had. It helped me forge a regular meditation practice and take up yoga, which I had wanted to do for years. Kris Carr has said she wouldn't call cancer a gift because she wouldn't choose to give it to anyone else, but she does label it a blessing. I do too.

Heather Swift, an ovarian and breast cancer survivor, said, "I have learned to make better choices. I wasn't always in healthy relationships. There were a number of ways in which I didn't know myself and didn't value myself. Didn't honor my own deep-seated needs to be who I am. Cancer taught me to look at my own needs and desires. I definitely feel that I approach things differently now. I would have eventually figured it out in some different ways," she said, "but cancer sped up the process."

Lynn Lane, founder of Voices of Survivors, said, "I learned how precious life is. All the things we think are important pretty much aren't. Pursue what's really meaningful," he said. "I was living an insane life before, and cancer really helped me let go of the material things—money, fame, etc.—and focus on what was really important. Art, photography and my family are what mean the most to me. When I talk about my life, it's post-cancer, not pre-cancer. It's kind of like being reborn and woken up. This is more of who I am."

Aileen said, "I create the kind of space that helps people be creative. I'm a muse," she said. "I would never have recognized that without cancer. A friend told me that I had really inspired her. She just loved me and saw things in me that I didn't see in myself."

Lesley said making big decisions about her life was always a challenge to her even before cancer, and afterward, she would wonder when starting something new if she would be around to see it completed. She says, "One of the 'gifts' cancer has given me is a pretty substantial ability to stay in the present where I let those dreary thoughts float away and not take up space in my body, heart and mind."

What is most important to you?

How has cancer changed your life for the better?

The New Normal

> *Nobody realizes that some people expend tremendous*
> *energy merely to be normal.*
> —ALBERT CAMUS

> *My whole life I wanted to be normal. Everybody knows*
> *there's no such thing as normal. There is no black-and-white*
> *definition of normal. Normal is subjective.*
> —TORI SPELLING

Many cancer survivors have said there is no longer any such thing as "normal," that we must get accustomed to a new normal. That idea makes a lot of sense to me. Cancer brings gifts as well as hardships, and for most of us, our lives will never be the same. For some, survival brings a new lease on life, the end to a destructive relationship they didn't have the courage to leave before, or the advent of a new passion to explore—personally or professionally. For others, it brings only surgery scars, early onset menopause, and depression. Most of us probably have some combination of both the blessings and the difficulties.

The end of treatment can often be the most challenging time of a cancer diagnosis, which is next to impossible for people in your life to understand. As caregivers and friends have supported you through the ravages of treatment, they are ready to celebrate its completion. You breathe a sigh of relief that it's over as well, and immediately following ask, "Now what?" While your friends, coworkers, and family members now expect your life to get back to normal immediately, you no longer have any idea what normal is. Almost universally, cancer survivors will tell you to get to know your "new normal."

The shock of diagnosis is followed by the long trudge through treatment, and for those with stage four disease, the slog never ends. Managing treatments for the rest of your life becomes the new normal. For the rest of us who have put our heads down and done what needed to be done, the end of treatment can be scary. No longer actively battling our disease, and consumed with managing side effects of treatment, fears about whether or not it worked begin to make their way into our minds.

While our environment calls for us to get back in the swing of things, we are still dealing with a variety of issues, such as no hair, neuropathy, lack of focus ("chemo brain"), and deep uncertainty about our disease and our lives. This can leave us feeling ungrounded and confused. A part of us wants to jump for joy, and another part is utterly stymied about what is next, and not sure where to turn for help.

Life is not the same following cancer treatment, and there are both upsides and drawbacks to that state of affairs. First and foremost, we can celebrate the fact that we have graduated to a new stage of the process that requires follow-up but less intense or no active treatment. Secondly, we can cultivate a deeper appreciation for life and what it now means to us. We have survived—with some scars, both physical and psychological, but relatively intact.

Many people proclaim that cancer has given them a new perspective on life, a deeper appreciation for the many blessings and gifts, and stronger connections with those they love. For those of us who are single, it can also make us feel very alone. It was difficult for me to go from being the center of attention when I was in treatment to being alone again as those who supported me began to fade into the background following the immediate crisis. Suddenly, all the attention, assistance, and connection that came along with treatment may not be as present, and that can be very lonely.

"Feeling all alone with my family so far away was the hardest part," one survivor shared. "I felt forced to take care of all issues by myself and often wouldn't tell other people what was happening because I didn't want to be a burden."

Pay particular attention to your feelings during this time, and communicate your needs to those around you. This is a good time to reach out to a mentor, counselor, or supportive friend to talk about what you are feeling. A social worker or navigator through your hospital or doctor's office can be helpful now as these individuals have seen this before with other patients and know what to expect.

"The biggest issue I see survivors struggle with," says Dr. Bolte, "is how to make sense of the experience. Not necessarily why it happened, but what do I want to do about it or with it. A cancer diagnosis can provide an opportunity for people to do things differently or reevaluate what they do or don't want out of life, relationships, career, etc."

Far from being over, your journey, in many ways, is just beginning. You have your whole life stretching out before you, but absolutely no idea of what it will look like now. The beauty is that you get to choose.

Try This
Now What

1. Make a list of the ways that you are different now than before your diagnosis. Acknowledge the difficult parts of this list and appreciate all the ways you are stronger.

2. Think about what you have always wanted to do—those dreams you've been putting off. Now is the time! Make a bucket list, life to-do list, or vision board. Put it somewhere you can see it daily.

3. Journal about what scares you, what you're uncertain about, and what you still need from your support network. Ask your doctor any questions you have about what's next. Talk to your friends and family, and let them know that your journey isn't quite finished. Talk to your mentor, coach, therapist, or other counselor about how you're feeling.

4. Cut yourself some slack. You don't have to jump into the deep end of your life right away. Wade in slowly, and give yourself some time to ramp back up to previous activity levels, OR NOT. Remember, *you* get to choose what your life looks like now.

Survivorship

Cancer changes your life, often for the better. You learn what's
important, you learn to prioritize, and you learn not to
waste your time. You tell people you love them. My friend Gilda Radner
(who died of ovarian cancer in 1989 at age 42) used to say, 'If it
wasn't for the downside, having cancer would be the
best thing and everyone would want it.' That's true.
If it wasn't for the downside.
—JOEL SIEGEL

Oh, my friend, it's not what they take away from you that counts—it's
what you do with what you have left.
—HUBERT HUMPHREY

Survivorship is a relatively new term in our collective vocabulary. It represents both a positive direction in medical advancements, and at the same time, a host of new long-term impacts from conventional cancer treatments as people are living longer with the disease. Many people are confused about what to call themselves or others when they are diagnosed with cancer. If you just found out yesterday that you have the disease, are you a survivor today? I say, absolutely, yes! Surviving the diagnosis is nothing to sneeze at, and those initial days can truly be the most difficult part—emotionally, if not physically. Wrapping your head around the idea that your life is now changed forever is no small task. Staring your mortality in the face is scary.

Being a survivor and living strong are empowering. Wouldn't you rather be called a survivor than a cancer patient or, worse, victim? We can

---

Keep Asking for Help

Having cancer is scary, and feeling alone with it when those worries come in the middle of the night and there is no one there to talk to about it, can definitely compound those fears. Reaching out and asking for help can feel like weakness; like admitting we can't do it all ourselves. Guess what? We can't. It is actually a show of your greatest strength to be able to ask for what you need. You may feel like the end of treatment signals the end of your needs. It doesn't. Asking for help is one of the most difficult things you will have to do, and you have to do it over and over again.

borrow some wisdom from the arenas of sexual assault or other forms of abuse. Being a survivor rather than a victim is always preferable. The minute you receive the diagnosis, you are surviving cancer, and every day you keep on breathing after that, you will be a survivor.

I met a pediatric neurological oncologist at a 4th of July party days before I was scheduled to begin chemo. In addition to pumping him for information about my chemo drugs and what kind of side effects I could expect, I shared my awe that he could do his job day in and day out. "Working with kids who have brain cancer must be so hard," I said. "Actually," he replied, "it's way better than 20 years ago when I started—many of the kids actually survive now."

Medicine really has come a long way. Many of those kids are experiencing side effects later in life from the therapies used to treat their illness, but at least they are alive.

Mihir is one of them. He was born with cancer, and has struggled with a variety of health issues his entire life as a result. At one point he was legally blind, and one of the chemo drugs he was given as a child has had long-term effects, causing his heart to fail when he was 24. After a pacemaker and other treatments, he finally got a heart transplant at 34. "I was lucky," he said. "Two months after going on the transplant list, I had a donor."

He considers himself extremely fortunate in other ways as well, and believes that lots of people are a lot worse off than him. "I have to do the best with what I've got," he says. "Why would I want to hurt those around me by being upset? Complaining isn't going to change anything." He feels that because he was given a heart, he owes it to the donor and the donor's family to make the most of his life. "If people could learn something from me, it would be to appreciate what you have."

Survivorship brings up a whole host of new issues for us to focus on, such as fertility concerns, long-term side effects of treatment, emotional issues, and financial ones too. These are good problems to have because they mean that the "patient" is still alive to have them. The medical establishment is recognizing more and more that each patient is not just a complaint or a disease, but a whole person with needs beyond the eradication of an illness.

I am proud to be a survivor, and whatever issues I have to deal with pale when measured against more time with my family and friends, important work to do, writing something that might help someone else going through a challenge, and great adventures and travel to experience. I appreciate all the joys, and sorrows too, of life. Everyone has survived something difficult, some of us much more than others. All experiences are valid and worthwhile, no matter how great or small. It's not the challenges we are given that matter. It's what we do with them.

What does the term "survivor" mean to you?

When did you consider yourself to be one?

How has your perspective on life changed since your diagnosis?

Beyond Surviving

> *All that is really necessary for survival of the fittest, it seems, is an interest in life, good, bad or peculiar.*
> —GRACE PALEY

> *Because our choices are largely based on survival. But if life is eternal, life is not a question.*
> —NEALE DONALD WALSH

Human beings are designed to survive. Our instincts guide us in fight or flight or other responses needed to survive whatever situation we find ourselves in. On one side of the coin, this is a comforting thought—survival is the norm, and we will take action instinctively when our safety and well-being is threatened. It is nice to know we don't have to stop and think in the face of danger, but just trust our instincts. But in another sense, "surviving" is kind of a mediocre standard to set for our lives.

Some of my cancer survivor friends question the widespread use of the term "survivor" as somewhat limiting. Hmmmm. I had never thought of it that way. While survivorship can be empowering, it isn't always. When you are fighting for your life, surviving is certainly optimal, but once the immediate danger has passed, don't we all yearn for something more?

It is so easy to become complacent in life, accepting the challenges as they come, and "surviving" on a day-to-day basis. It reminds me of the first line from the book *Good to Great* by Jim Collins, "Good is the enemy of great." So many of us settle for good, when our lives could be great, even extraordinary! Why? Because we are designed to survive. Taking the chance, as the lyrics to the Sugarland song "Something More" mention, entails risk, and that could threaten our survival. At the very least, it feels dangerous to step outside the comfortable box we have created for ourselves.

My cancer diagnosis freed me in so many ways from needing the stability and security I had previously pursued. Once you face your own mortality, and recognize that there is really no such thing as security in life, you realize that taking the risk to do something new can be the most rewarding part of your brief existence. This is true even if you fail miserably. After all, you will survive.

I am drawing on the wisdom of many others here, but why would I try to say it better than George Bernard Shaw did:

> This is the true joy in life. . .being used for a purpose recognized by yourself as a mighty one. . .being a force of Nature instead of a feverish selfish little clod of ailments and grievances complaining that the world will not devote itself to making you happy.
>
> . . .I am of the opinion that my life belongs to the whole community and as long as I live it is my privilege to do for it whatever I can. I want to be thoroughly used up when I die. For the harder I work the more I live. I rejoice in life for its own sake. Life is no brief candle to me. It's a sort of splendid torch, which I've got to hold up for the moment, and I want to make it burn as brightly as possible before handing it on to future generations.

Most of us are so afraid to live this way. In fact, we are afraid of everything: snakes, lightning, rapists, terrorists, tornadoes, embarrassment, failure, success, vulnerability. I'm not suggesting that these things aren't scary, only that they will be there whether we spend time being afraid of them or not.

Sean Swarner reacted powerfully to his diagnosis. Surviving two different forms of cancer as a teenager, he went away to college and largely created a new identity, partying and having fun, keeping his past illness on the down-low, and happy to no longer be known as "cancer boy." When it came time to find a job after graduation, Sean quickly realized that a typical 9 to 5 life wasn't for him. He decided to climb Mount Everest on behalf of other cancer survivors, despite the fact that he had never climbed a mountain before, had only half his normal lung capacity due to his treatment, and didn't have any financial backing or experienced guidance.

Sean and his brother packed their stuff in the car and drove to Colorado to start learning about mountains. Camping at first and then trading handyman services for lodging, Sean would climb local 14ers (peaks above 14,000 feet) during the day—eventually with 50 to 100 pounds of rocks in his pack—and in the afternoons, he would call potential sponsors to fund his trip. Eventually raising enough money to finance the very expensive expedition, Sean headed for Everest base camp. He didn't join an expedition with a large support team, but just hired a Sherpa to get him to the summit. His incredible story is told in the book *Keep Climbing: How I Beat Cancer and Reached the Top of the World*, co-written by Rusty Fischer.

This story isn't about how great Sean is, though he is. It is about how powerfully he responded to his circumstances. Sean didn't have a clue what he was doing when he began his quest to climb Mount Everest, and that is what makes it so extraordinary. He just set an intention and began taking what steps he saw in front of him to take. Literally one step at a time, the same way he eventually got up the mountain. Most of us have probably wanted to do something and told ourselves that we didn't know the right people, didn't have the money, the time, the knowledge to make it happen. Next time you have that thought, I hope you will remember this: Sean didn't either.

Living beyond surviving entails taking risks, but it offers tremendous rewards in return. Surviving is certainly better than the alternative, but what about something more?

What could you risk to gain something more?

If you believe that anything is possible—who will you be?

What are your wildest dreams (not just those that you think are achievable, but what you really yearn for)?

5

You Are Worthy

*When we see persons of worth, we should think of equaling
them; when we see persons of a contrary character,
we should turn inwards and examine ourselves.*
—CONFUCIUS

*The fact that you're struggling doesn't make you a burden.
It doesn't make you unlovable or undesirable or undeserving
of care. It doesn't make you too much or too sensitive or too needy.
It makes you human. Everyone struggles. Everyone has a difficult
time coping, and at times, we all fall apart. . .
The truth is that you can be struggling and still be loved.
You can be difficult and still be cared for.
You can be less than perfect, and still be deserving
of compassion and kindness.*
—DANIELL KOEPKE

You are worthy of whatever you desire for yourself and your life: a comfortable home, a fulfilling career, financial abundance, a loving relationship. As Wayne Dyer says, "Self-worth comes from one thing—thinking that you are worthy."

I have struggled with believing I was inherently worthy of whatever I wanted. Intellectually, I knew I wasn't worthless. I knew I was valuable and valued. I just didn't fully believe in my own worth, and on top of that, I wasn't even aware there was anything about this floating around in my subconscious.

Only when I finally began to recognize how my own worthiness issues manifest could I begin to address them. For example, I used to give more than I received, believing people would only like me if I was helpful and giving. I didn't feel that just being me and showing up was enough. Sure, I have always been independent and self-sufficient, but the underlying reasons were that I didn't believe I was worthy of others' time or attention or help. I didn't want to be a bother to anyone.

We are all whole, complete, and perfect as we are. We don't have to work on ourselves or fix or change anything about ourselves to be worthy. Just the very fact that we exist means we are worthy to receive love, money, kindness, friendship, or anything we desire.

Worthy of Connection

As I read through the responses to my survey of single people who have had cancer, one theme resonated loud and clear through nearly all of them: a feeling that we are somehow unworthy now of being loved. We are damaged goods, have scars and fewer body parts, might not be able to have children, might relapse and die, lost our hair, our dignity, our sense of self. These feelings are common and very real to those of us who have been through this journey. Being a single cancer survivor can be a double-whammy, because being without a partner may already cause us to wonder why we can't seem to find a mate when so many others have, and we may think, "What is wrong with me?" Consciously, most of us know that this thought is complete nonsense, but subconsciously we can sabotage ourselves by thinking this way and create a self-fulfilling prophecy.

In a workshop with single cancer survivors a few years ago I asked the participants what "single" meant to them. The answers were: loser, alone, lonely, and other similar words and phrases. Activists like Bella DePaulo, PhD, have written about how singles are "stereotyped, stigmatized and ignored." Her book *Singled Out* details the ways in which singles are discriminated against in our society (the single supplement on many trips and special event pricing for couples being just two small examples), the stereotypes we face, and the fact that we are often labeled as selfish.

As evidenced by the research about health and well-being, most of us should be more selfish with our time and attention, instead of spending so much time trying to please others or society. Personally, "selfish" was always the worst thing I could be called, though mostly that label came from myself, and I did everything I could to avoid appearing so in any way. I regularly repressed my own desires to please the group, gave up my time to things I felt I should do rather than really wanting to, and didn't set clear boundaries for myself.

DePaulo also suggests that "family values" have been bastardized to leave out the vast majority of us who are raising kids as single parents, living alone, or even part of same sex couples. Singles often even pay higher tax rates, despite the so-called "marriage penalty" we hear so much about in the media. All of this reinforces the feeling many of us have that something must be wrong with us if we're single. We live in a society that values couplehood, but more and more of us are remaining single much longer these days, and more people live alone than at any time in our history.

For single cancer survivors, the stigma can be doubly or triply painful as infertility issues, scars, and other body image issues, the specter of illness, and fear of recurrence all combine to make us wonder who could possibly love us now? Some of us believe our past illness makes us somehow unworthy or undeserving of love, and we sometimes wallow in self-pity, which does actually make us less desirable.

The truth is that all of us are whole and complete and worthy of love no matter what we have dealt with in our past. We all have something to offer, and a beautiful spirit to share with others, even if we are missing a breast, ovaries, a testicle, a limb, or have physical and emotional scars from the experience of life and illness. It is truly only our own limitations that hold us back and keep us from sharing the love in our hearts.

The Physical and Psychological Scars of Cancer

I realized something quite shocking about my relationships post-cancer, and while now the pattern seems so obvious, for three years I didn't see it. I said all the things to myself that you may have said to yourself: I am unattractive, unworthy, and unlovable. At the end of chemo when I looked and felt my worst—bald, overweight, no eyebrows or lashes, zits—I felt so undesirable. I told myself I couldn't date again until I had hair and had gotten back into reasonable shape, and I didn't.

Eventually, my body recovered, my hair grew back, the zits went away, and my weight returned to normal when I stopped taking the steroids that go along with chemo. But for a long time my psyche didn't. Those feelings of unattractiveness and unworthiness were lurking beneath the surface. It didn't seem to matter that I looked as good or better than I had before treatment; that I was working out with a trainer, and in great shape; that my hair had grown back as full and thick as before and that others were complimenting me. Inside, I still must have felt undesirable; otherwise, I wouldn't have acted the way I did.

For three years I only dated men I liked and enjoyed talking to but wasn't attracted to, or on the flip side, had purely sexual relationships, even meaningless hookups that I never would have had before. At the time, I wasn't embarrassed or ashamed of these hookups at all. They were what I needed, I reasoned, and I enjoyed them. I even told myself that perhaps this was better than a long-term relationship—easier, less complicated, and more fun.

That was the case until one relationship came crashing down around me, and I finally recognized what was going on. I met him after an intense weekend together in a leadership program. He went away for two weeks right afterward, during which we texted and occasionally talked on the phone. It seemed to take almost no time for the texts to become sexual in nature, and while I felt like things were moving too fast at times, it was also exciting. When he came back to town, he surprised me by showing up at my condo on a Saturday afternoon, and he didn't leave until Monday morning.

That set the pattern for the rest of our time together—long weekends spent largely in bed, sexy texts when we were away from each other (which was fairly often), and a lot of fun but little substance. I knew he only related to me in a sexual way, and while it occasionally bothered me, for the most part, I reveled in it. He loved my body and told me so often, brought me out of my shell in many ways, and taught me to appreciate many new things I hadn't tried before.

It wasn't until four months in that I discovered he had also met another woman in the same leadership program the same weekend he met me, and had also been seeing her the entire time. The difference was, he had told her he loved her, and they had been planning a life together and talking about marriage. Though I didn't know it, I was the "other woman," the one he was just having sex with. That made it both easier in some ways and more difficult in others. I wasn't as emotionally invested, so it wasn't as devastating to me, but I also wondered why I wasn't the one he fell in love with.

This scenario could have easily sent me into my same old patterns of feeling unworthy, less than, and unlovable. Ironically, the same leadership program where he and I met helped equip me to see things differently this time. The most difficult and most important step in this process was to take responsibility for my role in the situation—not the cheating, but the relationship I had co-created with him. I not only accepted a sexual relationship, I loved it. It made me feel sexy and desirable, and I had so much fun. Being with him validated me.

Realizing this is what enabled me to see the pattern of those three post-chemo years. Three of the men I had been with during that time had been in love with someone else. I didn't know that when I was with them, but clearly my feelings of not being desirable were attracting men who only wanted to hook up with me. It would be easy to make them wrong, marvel at how gross they were, and stop trusting people, but all I really have control over is me. I have the power to change me, and how I relate to people.

I am ashamed of how I behaved during that time, and I share it because it is the most real and authentic example I can give of the damage we do to ourselves. Landmark Education taught me that we all have the ability to live life powerfully and live a life we love. That is both a comforting and a terrifying thought. If I can create any possibility for myself and my life that I want, then I have to take full responsibility for doing that. I can no longer blame other people or my circumstances or my schedule or anything else for not getting what I desire. In order to get what I want, I first have to believe I'm worthy of it.

To prove the truth in that, I want to share what happened with this particular situation. The "other woman" and I both realized we were selling ourselves short and accepting less than we were worthy of. We became good friends, supported each other through the early, painful part of the break-up, and communicated nearly every day for a while. We also both forgave him and remain friendly with him. It was very powerful to be able to respond to a painful situation this way. And because we didn't attack him and make him wrong, he didn't have to be defensive and could go straight to taking responsibility for his part. He recognized a pattern of selfishness and egomania extending to several past relationships, and even called his ex-wife to apologize for his role in the dissolution of their marriage.

Now I realize what I am worthy of, and I'm not willing to settle for less. I attract amazing men into my life. They aren't necessarily beating down my door, but the quality (if not the quantity) of my relationships is very different from those initial post-chemo years. I know when I am fully ready for him, the right guy will show up, and until then, I can enjoy dating.

Recently, I met a man I was sure was the perfect person for me. The way it played out showed me that I was absolutely acting from a place of worthiness. There were numerous signs, fortuitous timing, we had similar values and beliefs—this was it. I was sure of it, and I was so excited! Only, . . . he wasn't sure. As we got to know each other better, I could tell he was also struggling with issues of worthiness and was scared to really allow himself to love someone.

Because I had been there, I wanted to help him deal with his own stuff. It was so obvious to me on the other side of it how we push away whatever we feel we aren't worthy of. No matter how much I loved him, he couldn't let it in. What a powerful mirror for my own experience. I wanted to help him overcome his issues, but mainly so he could love me. I realized I definitely wasn't OK with investing my own time and energy to "help" only to have him fall in love with someone else.

I had been convinced that it wasn't that he didn't love me, it was that he wasn't capable of loving anyone, or really receiving the love offered to him. That may or may not be the case, but what I finally realized was that I was worthy of someone who could love me fully and completely. I didn't need to help or convince or cajole someone into it. The right person just would.

He and I are still really close. We are great friends and talk regularly, and he is a total blessing in my life. I no longer carry around any frustration that our relationship isn't what it could be, I just appreciate it for what it is. The best part is that I am standing very firmly in my own worthiness to be adored, beloved, and wooed.

While my scars were hidden and psychological, Leah's were visible and physical. At 26 she was diagnosed with papillary carcinoma after several years of signs that something was wrong. Surgeons removed not only her thyroid, but 40 lymph nodes, three of four parathyroids, and a good amount of muscle from her neck, leaving her with a thick line of scar tissue painted like an ear-to-ear necklace.

The scar was a painful reminder to Leah every time she looked in the mirror, and she made efforts to cover it up whenever possible. She wondered, "Who could ever be attracted to someone that has this hideous scar on her neck?" and felt as if she had to tell her story on every first date because it was so obvious that something had happened.

Turtlenecks became a safe haven for her, until covering and hiding the scar felt as heavy a burden as the scar itself. She felt ashamed, until she realized she could learn to become more comfortable with both her diagnosis and the physical reminders of it. She began to see it instead as a great opportunity to share, which she was surprised to learn released her anxiety about it. Eventually, the scar became a part of her healing process, and a reminder, not of her brokenness, but of her strength.

One man said, "I still struggle with what to tell anybody I meet, especially women I'm romantically interested in, about my medical history. I had a scar revision to replace my original thyroidectomy scar that looked like something on Frankenstein's monster. Even though the new scar is fading, I'm still conscious of it everyday, and I make sure it's covered up by whatever shirt I wear."

I love the sex scene in *Lethal Weapon 3* that begins with Mel Gibson and Rene Russo comparing scars from their many years of police work. They peel off layer after layer of clothing in an escalating attempt to one-up the other about who has the best scar. Like it or not, we all have emotional and physical scars from life—as cancer survivors perhaps more so than the general population, but likely less so than some war veterans. What if they didn't have to be painful reminders or something to be embarrassed about? What if we could summon up some pride instead for what we have survived, and know that we are absolutely worthy of being loved despite our battle wounds?

What are some times in your life when you devalued your own worth?

What can you take responsibility for in those situations?

What do you value the most about yourself?

You Are Enough

In her book *Daring Greatly*, Brene Brown writes that the opposite of scarcity is not abundance. It is enough. I am enough. You are enough. Most pain comes from comparing ourselves to others and finding something lacking, but our inherent worth is in just being authentically who we really are. There is no one else exactly like you on the planet, and if you aren't you, then whatever you have to contribute and create won't exist. If someone doesn't love you for who you are, then he or she isn't worthy of being in your life.

Dying to Be Me is the autobiography of Anita Moorjani. During a near death experience caused by her organs shutting down from late stage cancer, she discovered a profound truth about life: that we are all here to be ourselves, experience joy and love, and recognize the connection of all living things. Our biggest fear is that we are disconnected and separate. This is actually the definition of shame according to Brown, a researcher and author from the University of Houston. Her famous TED Talks explore the importance of vulnerability and its link to shame. She says shame is the feeling that there is something about us that makes us unworthy of being connected or loved, and when we feel that way, we are less likely to be open and vulnerable with others, which creates more separation and disconnection.

We all vacillate between two states of being, according to Brown: "never good enough" on the one hand, and, if we manage to overcome that, "who do you think you are?" She says the courage to be imperfect, show compassion to ourselves, and let go of who we "should be" in order to be who we are allows us to be authentically ourselves, and that sharing ourselves openly and vulnerably is what makes us beautiful. Her research interviewing hundreds of people has pointed to one truth: that the people who have a strong sense of love and belonging are those who believe they are worthy of it. Period.

Try This
Affirmations

Affirmations are statements we can use to envision our desired future and affirm, or cement, something in the present. They are especially powerful if recited while looking in the mirror and into your own eyes. For this reason, you may want to post them on a sticky note onto your bathroom mirror to remind yourself to do them once or twice a day, though the more you do them, the more powerfully they will be cemented for you. A simple one to start with is: I am enough. Repeat it several times to allow it to really sink in. Some of my current affirmations are:

- I am responsible for my life. I can handle any situation.
- There is plenty of love, work, and money for everyone.
- I am abundant with love, trust, and support.
- I love myself, body and soul.

What do you want to affirm for yourself each day? Write 5 to 10 of your own affirmations and post them somewhere that you will see them every day. I have one on my bedroom ceiling, right above my bed, so it is the last thing I see before I close my eyes, and the first thing I see when I wake up.

I wrote an Enough Manifesto as an assignment from a business coach who helped me recognize that my natural gift is in seeing and valuing people for who they really are. Part of sharing my gifts is recognizing my own "enoughness," or worthiness to do so. You can read it on pages 173 and 175 and download a color poster version from the website IAmTracyMaxwell.com.

Try This

Write Your Own Manifesto

It doesn't have to follow the same format as mine, or even adhere to the subject of being enough. Make it your own.

Answer these questions:

- Who are you?
- Who do you want to be?
- What do you believe in?
- What do you know to be true (for you)?
- What makes life worth living?
- What makes you feel the most? (laugh, smile, cry, jump for joy)

CHAPTER

6

You Are Lovable

If you want to be loved, be lovable.
—OVID

*At the heart of personality is the need to feel a sense of being
lovable without having to qualify for that acceptance.*
—PAUL TOURNIER

*Self-esteem is made up primarily of two things: feeling lovable
and feeling capable.*
—JACK CANFIELD

We all need love, affection, attention, intimacy, and camaraderie, and those things are always available to us. When are the times you are most likely to seek them out? Is it only when you are having a rough time? Do people seem more likely to provide them when things are really at their worst? This kind of pattern could cause us to subconsciously create situations that allow us to be supported in ways that we aren't normally.

What is your reaction to hearing the phrase, "You are whole, complete, and perfect just as you are"? Do you believe that? Or does your ego instantly throw back all the reasons you aren't? We all sometimes feel as if we need to be fixed in some way, that if we could just look this way or have that skill or do that thing that we value, we would be worthy of that dream job, relationship, or home. The truth is that you don't have to do anything to be worthy of love. You just are.

I said this to someone I was dating once. I told him he was whole, perfect, complete, and worthy of being loved right now. "How do I know this?" I asked him. "Because I love you." I have chosen many men who didn't think they were worthy of me. They were a mirror for my own issues. The things that bother you the most about others? Look at yourself. Something similar is probably lurking around in there. If we don't feel lovable, we can't really allow anyone else to love us.

Dating, sex, fertility, and marriage are all likely topics that produce a certain amount of anxiety for you, as they did for me and many of the single survivors I spoke with in writing this book. It doesn't have to be that way, if you learn to really embrace your own lovability. When you know you are lovable, you don't take it personally when you get rejected by someone. You recognize instead that it's not about you. The right person, at the right time, will love you no matter what.

Try This
You Are Lovable

Take out a journal or piece of paper and write down all the things that are lovable about you. E-mail 10 friends and ask them what they love about you. Call your parents and siblings or other family members and ask them what they love most about you. If you are feeling especially brave, reach out to past romantic partners and ask them what they appreciated, liked, or loved most about you.

Wabi-Sabi

No matter how many things are on the list of lovable things, or how many people supplied them, you may be saying to yourself, yeah, but this part of me is never going to be lovable. This scar or flaw or bad habit or body part is just not lovable. And even that is not true, my friend. Sometimes the parts of ourselves that we dislike the most are exactly the parts that someone else loves.

The term "wabi-sabi" represents a Japanese aesthetic about the acceptance of imperfection. It is derived from Buddhist teachings, and often applied to art that is flawed in some way—a cracked vase, a disproportional painting, and so on. Wabi-sabi is used to describe beauty that is "imperfect, impermanent, and incomplete." Basically, wabi-sabi suggests that it is exactly those parts of us we find most flawed that can be endearing to others.

I once began an online dating profile by disclosing that I was a total klutz who could "trip on a pattern in the carpeting." My friend asked me if I was sure I wanted to lead with this negative. I decided to keep it because, to me, it was so honest. I had more responses to that profile than any I have ever posted, as men responded to me sharing their own stories of klutziness. One said, "I tripped walking across the stage to receive my high school diploma," whereas another shared, "I cut myself shaving this morning."

Usually, dating profiles list only what we feel makes us most desirable, and we post the best photo ever taken of us, but this isn't reality. We don't always look that way, and there is more to us than our love of long walks on the beach, no matter how great that may sound at first read. What if we could appreciate all the parts of us instead, even those that we think of as weakness, flawed, or just plain human?

We look at others and get intimidated by the fact that they are so successful or good-looking or wealthy, and we use that status to put them on a pedestal and assume they are somehow better than us. The truth is that each of those people once struggled, lost a job or important relationship, had zits, or went bankrupt, and we might be shocked to know what they are dealing with behind the perfect façade, even now. Knowing those struggles helps us relate to them in a more personal way.

Dating

> *I can't even find someone for a platonic relationship, much less*
> *the kind where someone wants to see me naked.*
> —GILBERT GOTTFRIED

> *I don't know the first real thing about the dating game. I don't know how*
> *to talk to a specific person and connect. I just think you have to go person*
> *by person, and do the best you can with people in general.*
> —JASON SCHWARTZMAN

"At what point in a new relationship is it appropriate to reveal your status as a cancer survivor?" I posed this question to my friend who is HIV positive. His situation is perhaps a bit more relevant in a dating relationship because of the sexual implications of his disease. His answer was that every situation is different, and that I would just have to do what feels natural in each case. I never have trouble revealing my cancer status to new friends or even total strangers. It just seems to come out, and it's not something I have anxiety about anymore. However, many survivors ask this question in relation to sharing with potential romantic partners.

Advice from other survivors varies. Some say do it right away before things get too serious, so if the person bolts, you aren't emotionally invested. Others insist it's better to wait until you know there's a future before sharing because there's no point putting yourself out there that way if there's not. For those of us who are really open about our status and/or work in the cancer advocacy arena, we don't usually have to worry about it because these days anyone who does an Internet search for us will already know. My favorite advice comes from Tamika, who says to share with someone only when they are worthy of knowing: when you know you like them enough to see a possibility, but before things get too serious and they feel like you withheld something important from them.

Collin, a 27-year-old testicular cancer survivor from Chicago, said, "It usually comes up naturally when I talk about my volunteer work with Imerman Angels in the first three to four dates. If it doesn't," he says, "then it is around our first sexual experience when I have to explain the prosthetic testicle."

Jasan, a three-time cancer survivor living in Palo Alto, California, had a bad experience with one woman after he disclosed his cancer history, which he said made him more nervous about his reveal afterward. He heard Kairol Rosenthal speak, and she said somewhere between the third and fifth date is the ideal time to tell. Her book, *Everything Changes*, details her own cancer experience and that of several other young adult survivors.

Jasan is married now. He met his wife online and they dated for nearly two years before getting engaged. She said, "He was nervous to tell me because of responses he had gotten in the past. But I told him, 'I'm not a shallow bitch. That's not going to scare me away.'" Even though her mom died when she was 13 and her dad is a cancer survivor, Jen says cancer isn't going to make her not want to be with someone.

Single Survivor Stats

85% said they felt anxiety or inadequacy about dating.

83% said body image issues were a major concern.

By the time I had at least 2 to 3 inches of hair back, I decided I looked normal enough to not have to deal with questions on the first date, and I put myself out there. I started trolling the personals on Craigslist—a first for me. I have done the online dating thing before, but always the services that required payment. Often, I had been overwhelmed by the number of incoming e-mails. This time, I decided to do the choosing myself rather than wading through responses from men.

I try to put myself in their position. How would I have reacted if someone I was dating told me he had cancer? I'm sure I would wonder how long he's going to be around, and whether it's worth getting involved with someone who may have a shorter life expectancy and may well get sick again. It's one thing if you're already in love with someone who gets sick, but would you choose to get involved with that scenario?

There are plenty of reasons that guys have rejected me in the past, do we really want to add cancer to the list? I will never forget my Grandma's advice—she was a nurse—when I mentioned in high school that I had a crush on this guy who had diabetes. She ran down all the problems related to that chronic disease, and told me I would be better off liking someone else.

Heather Hall could identify with this as well. One guy she dated was thrilled to find out she was a survivor too, and would understand. "I got nervous," she said, "because he had cancer three times. I couldn't stop thinking about what if we had kids. I thought, really?! I'm such a hypocrite! But I know what it's like. I lost my dad to cancer and had it myself. I work for a cancer organization. I'm too close to it."

Heather was diagnosed with osteosarcoma her senior year of college at age 21. She currently serves as the executive director of Gilda's Club in Detroit, and recently got married. She also struggled with how to tell people. "Sometimes I would just tell them about the knee," she said of her new titanium parts. "I mention that I had it replaced and leave it at that." One guy broke up with her the day after she revealed her status. He had lost three family members to cancer and said he couldn't go through that again. "I was offended at first because I'm not going to die of cancer. But then I totally understood from his point of view."

Some survivors have had positive experiences dating after cancer. Brian, a 32-year-old gay survivor, said, "People think I'm strong, and rather than shy away, they seem to admire me. This experience changed me and I really feel comfortable with who I am now. I used to have so much anxiety." He also believes there is more compassion in the gay community because of AIDS.

Lesley, a breast cancer survivor from Colorado, said she was pursued during treatment even when she didn't have hair and added, "I think this has made me a better, more appealing person. When I lost my hair and my breasts, I felt stripped down and raw. Oddly enough, I gained a self-confidence I didn't have before. Considering I run a nonprofit to empower and support other women, it usually comes up pretty fast," she says. "I want to be with someone who isn't freaked out by it."

Lesley runs the Pink Elephant Posse, an organization that finds young women affected by cancer and puts them in the spotlight so their stories can be heard. Their mission is to inspire, empower, and connect survivors who may feel out of place—like a pink elephant—following cancer.

Lynn, a 44-year-old prostate cancer survivor and founder of Voices of Survivors, shared that his girlfriend is a two-time cancer survivor. "Cancer was actually more of a connection for us than a problem," he said. "I am really open about my status. Within five minutes of meeting me, you will know I had cancer."

Sean said after surviving two different deadly forms of childhood cancer he wasn't afraid to ask the most attractive girl for a date, because he didn't care if she said no. He was just happy to be alive, and didn't care what anyone thought about him. That fearlessness has stayed with him post-cancer as he climbs the tallest mountains in the world. But the one thing he was unsure of in the beginning was sharing his health history with the person he was dating. "There isn't a real opportune time to say, 'hey, by the way. . .I almost died a few years ago,'" Sean said.

In college, he explained, he did it awkwardly, playing dates a video of a television commercial that featured his inspirational story rather than telling them directly. Even though he asked them not to judge him and reminded them that he was still the same guy they already knew, he said the response was not usually great, and he figured he needed a new approach. Now he believes it shouldn't really matter. He suggests switching positions and considering how you would feel if someone you were dating told you they had had cancer. "Would you judge someone because of what happened to them in the past? You have someone who loves you, and you love that person back. Would it matter if they had been sick?"

While no one will probably ever list cancer on their Match.com profile—unless it's their astrological sign—it should be something we are comfortable talking about and dealing with. After all, more and more young adults are being diagnosed with cancer these days—there are 1 million survivors under 40 at last count. There is a whole movement serving this segment of the cancer population, and more awareness is being raised about the unique needs of this group. The myriad of dating issues I have mentioned will be faced by a significant segment of dating-age people in the future. I guess that means I need to practice my reveal, though at this point, I'm pretty sure the cat is out of the bag.

Relationships

> *Falling in love and having a relationship are two different things.*
> —KEANU REEVES

> *The worst relationship on earth is being in love with*
> *someone and still single.*
> —Meek Mill

As a single survivor in his twenties, Jonny Imerman, the well-known founder of Imerman Angels, dove into a relationship the second he finished treatment. "I just wanted my life back," he said. "I was happy to be alive and wanted someone in my life to anchor me. Life was all over the place and I was looking for stability."

In retrospect, that wasn't such a good approach as he realized that chemo Jonny was tired a lot and not that social. As he regained his famous energy and enthusiasm, the woman who was a perfect fit immediately following treatment—shy and more of a homebody—wasn't such a great match for the outgoing Imerman. When he experienced a blood clot and was in danger of possibly losing his arm he wasn't sure she could handle it.

"It was major. Really risky. It could have killed me. I remember her looking at me and telling me she didn't know if she could be with me if I had lost my arm. There is a threshold or breaking point for a lot of people at which it is just too much," Jonny says. "'Why sign up for this baggage when I can find someone who hasn't had cancer?' The task is to find people who are loyal and can take it; who love you no matter what."

Jonny advises the newly diagnosed and fresh out of treatment to temper their enthusiasm. He says he just wanted to catch up because he felt like he had missed so much time being sick. That feeling, coupled with the high of beating cancer, made him a bit hasty. He suggests getting your bearings again before making any big life decisions. Not just dating, but also moving or career decisions.

"Be excited about life," he says "but realize that you will be impulsive right after treatment. There is no rush."

Control vs. Surrender

Wanting to be in control is one way to protect yourself in relationships. This can manifest as controlling your emotions, what your dates are like (where we go, what we eat, how it will all play out, and when they will take place), and perhaps even planning out the entire relationship. We not only try to control ourselves, but our partners as well. We see all the things they are doing "wrong," and genuinely want to help them. When we point out these issues and offer "advice" though, we come off as nags, and send the message that our partner isn't good enough. This does not make for good romance.

Laura Doyle emphasizes in *The Surrendered Single* that our partners want us to be happy, and will do quite a bit to ensure our happiness. We don't have to manipulate or control to get what we want. We just have to ASK.

Overly Independent

An independent, "I can do it myself" attitude could be a turn off to potential partners, who often need to be needed. They want to help, and when they offer and we don't accept they feel snubbed. It doesn't mean they see us as weak and incapable, but just that they want to contribute to us. Adopting an independent attitude has served me well for many years in a variety of ways, but it has not helped in the romance department. If the man I'm dating needs to be needed, and I don't need any help, thank you very much, then where does that leave me?

Giving and Receiving

Does putting others' needs before our own make us better partners? Hmmm...maybe not. Turns out being a good receiver is pretty important too. If you are always giving and deflecting what others are offering, they aren't likely to keep giving to you.

Does this mean you shouldn't ever give anything in a relationship? Of course not. It's important to maintain a balance and allow yourself to receive more, while also perhaps giving differently—from a true desire, and not an unconscious effort to get people to like you or because you feel like you should. Giving so people will like us is manipulative and controlling, even if it is unconscious. Look at the motivations behind your giving. Are they selfless acts or is there an ulterior motive?

Vulnerability and Intimacy

We all think putting our best face forward is necessary in most parts of our lives. Think about the job interview, online dating profile, and résumé. We don't mention our weaknesses, fears, or flaws in these arenas. In most of life it is OK to talk about the less than perfect parts of ourselves, our insecurities, doubts, and mistakes. In fact, it's required if we want to have true intimacy.

We all have weaknesses, vulnerabilities, and things of which we are ashamed. Opening up about them gives others permission to do the same, and creates a new level of intimacy that probably wouldn't have been possible otherwise. This is what relating to each other is all about. And relating to someone else in a deeper way is what makes a relationship.

What are you trying to control in your relationships? How could you surrender instead?

What traits do you have that keep you separate from others?

What could you share that you are most ashamed of with someone you trust?

Touch

Let us touch the dying, the poor, the lonely and the unwanted according to the graces we have received and let us not be ashamed or slow to do the humble work.
—Mother Teresa

At the touch of love everyone becomes a poet.
—Plato

Studies in orphanages and hospitals stress that infants deprived of skin contact lose weight, become ill, and even die. To thrive, newborns need touch as much as food. As children, we instinctively seek out touch when we need it, and ask to be hugged or cuddled by our parents. As we grow older, we may not experience as much physical touch in our lives, and might not feel as comfortable asking for it. Nothing can make us feel loved more than being touched. A pat on the arm, a back rub, a hug, or someone stroking our hair all send the message, "I care about you." "You are loved." When we don't get this kind of physical contact, it can significantly contribute to feelings of loneliness and separation.

When I was going through cancer treatment, I had Reiki sessions once a week to help me deal with the side effects of chemo. This energy work from an ancient Japanese healing practice made a major impact on my nausea, bone aches, and physical issues. Looking back on it now, I also recognize how emotionally healing it was during that difficult time to receive loving touch for an hour each week.

Massage can help patients deal with lingering pain or sensitivity in certain body parts. It also helps move toxic chemicals out of the system, and provides a sense of rejuvenation to the body. But perhaps the most significant part of the process is the opportunity to talk with a provider about what you're going through as a patient or survivor, and to experience the connection that comes from allowing yourself to receive therapeutic touch.

Touch is one of *The 5 Love Languages* described by Gary Chapman in his popular series of books—there is even a version for singles. Chapman says that when our partner, friends, or family speak to us in our love language—the one that most resonates with us—we feel loved. Understandably, we tend to show others love the way we most appreciate receiving love, and that doesn't always strike the right chord. While all five approaches are important in loving relationships, one or two will click most strongly with each individual. They are: (1) touch, (2) quality time, (3) acts of service, (4) gifts, (5) affirmations.

My love language is definitely physical touch, followed closely by quality time. When I am dating someone and we are in close proximity, if we aren't touching in some way, holding hands, sitting close, cuddling, I feel as if something is wrong. I definitely feel most loved when physically connecting with someone else through hugs or other forms of physical affection and when spending quality time with that person doing something I enjoy.

When we are sick, people can be afraid they are going to hurt us in some way if they hug too hard or touch the wrong spot. This was the case for Brian, who said he barely received any human touch from family and friends during his treatment for stage IV non-Hodgkin's lymphoma at 29. As he described how traumatizing it was to be told you have advanced disease at such a young age, his voice broke several times.

"I was really scared of so many things," he said. "I wondered if I was going to die. Who was going to take care of me? About what was next. I barely take Tylenol," he admitted, "and I wondered if the chemo would kill me. I got two infections and was really sick. Everyone was afraid to touch me because of the three tubes coming out of my chest and the germ factor."

When we have ports, IVs, or other tubes and wires coming from our bodies, especially in the hospital, people can be even less willing to reach out physically. Let people know it's OK and where there might be sensitive areas to avoid. Go a step further and let your loved ones know when you need to hold someone's hand, or get an extra-long hug or a foot rub. Whatever makes you feel connected and loved—be willing to ask for it.

Being able to recognize your own needs and communicate them to others is essential. Saying to someone—whether they are a romantic partner, a friend, or family member— "Can you hold my hand?" can feel uncomfortable at first, but the more you practice it, the more natural it seems. "I like it when you rub my low back" is a great phrase to ensure you get more of what nurtures you. "Cuddling with you as we fall asleep is one of my favorite parts of the day" not only communicates what you like, but acknowledges the other person for what he or she gives to you.

Brian feels incredibly lucky that his mom cared for him during treatment and his entire family has been so supportive. His younger brother also had cancer, so unfortunately, they have experience with this sort of thing. "I'm a hugger," he says, "even though I worry about germs. I have always believed in the power of massage as well, and I get one once a month." He said he used to get deep tissue massage, and now he needs a much lighter touch because of the bone pain and the numerous needle biopsies he's had on his lower back. It's important to communicate with your practitioner about what intensity of pressure works for you.

I have used energy work such as Reiki, massage, and acupuncture to deal with many of the side effects of treatment and of menopause following my hysterectomy as well. All have had a profound impact on my physical issues, but perhaps just as strongly, if not more so, on my emotional well-being. The act of receiving is powerful, and all of these healing modalities ask only that you relax and allow yourself to receive the healing energy and touch being provided. There is something very profound about being able to receive in this way without any expectation of reciprocation. There are few times in our lives when we can do that.

Single people may not get as much affectionate touch as they need to feel healthy, connected, and loved. As society becomes less dependent upon each other for our physical survival, the emotional connections we have had with others historically have also fallen away. Just because we no longer need the community to hunt and kill our food, or to live collectively to share the tasks of daily survival, doesn't mean we are any less dependent upon each other for physical affection and companionship.

Living alone and being independent is becoming more and more common in modern society, and that can mean many of us are starved for human touch and affection. A friend was brave enough to share how difficult it was for him to have grown up without a great deal of affection in his home, and now, as a single adult, how isolating it can be to come home from a difficult day at work and not have someone to share that with or to give him a hug and let him know it is going to be OK.

His confession brought tears to my eyes because I often felt the same way going through cancer treatment. Not having someone there to help you make the difficult decisions that need to be made about your health and treatment can leave you feeling overwhelmed, but not having someone there to give you a hug and tell you everything's going to be OK is devastating. It may feel repetitive at this point, but I'm going to say it again: ask for what you need when you need it. Even if you have to call someone and say, "I need a hug. Can you come over?" Do that.

What kinds of physical affection do you crave that most comfort you?

How can you ask those in your life to give you the affectionate touch that you need?

Who will you reach out to for physical connection?

Sex

> *Sex is full of lies. The body tries to tell the truth. But it's usually too battered with rules to be heard, and bound with pretenses so it can hardly move. We cripple ourselves with lies.*
> —JIM MORRISON

> *Sex is emotion in motion.*
> —MAE WEST

Sex can be complicated under the best of circumstances, but following a cancer diagnosis, the complications multiply. Emotionally and physically, we aren't the same people we were before, and both sides of the sexual equation can be significantly impacted. Post-cancer bodies may not perform the same as before, and emotionally, we may be more fragile, uncertain, or even less connected.

Earlier, I shared my unconscious pattern of meaningless sexual experiences with a number of men who were in relationships. Even though I wasn't aware of the latter, I know that my own feelings of being undesirable attracted those situations. Tamika shared a similarly destructive dynamic in her relationships post-cancer. "I allowed men to be cruel to me," she said, "because that is what I thought I deserved."

After a cervical cancer diagnosis, Tamika had radiation and surgery to her vagina and is missing several inches of it as a result. She says she wanted to be the same person sexually and tried to be, but it didn't work. Some of her sexual partners were understanding and some weren't. Post-cancer, Tamika needed certain things to make sex pleasurable for her. That involved lubricants and more time and patience. When things weren't working, she told one partner she was sorry and perhaps they could try again later. His response was, "You're right. Try again. That's all we'll be doing. Trying." That's not love when someone treats you that way, Tamika said.

"No matter what, your body is never going to be the same," Tamika says. "It can be better or worse. It depends upon your perspective."

Tamika has been very open about her sexuality post-cancer as the founder of Tamika and Friends, a nonprofit dedicated to raising awareness about cervical cancer and its links to HPV. "Many people don't talk about this," Tamika said, "so I got over my own embarrassment and began to share, because it's important to me for others not to suffer this way in silence."

Cindy (not her real name) was diagnosed with ovarian cancer in high school, and it has impacted every area of her life ever since. While she is doing OK physically, and doesn't have enduring problems, she feels increasingly isolated, especially when it comes to dating and romance. She feels as if she never matured beyond high school emotionally. "I have always been sexually repressed," she admitted. "I'm Catholic and went to Catholic high school where I was focused on my studies and didn't really date."

She describes going through puberty as difficult, and said she was uncomfortable with her body changing. When she had ovarian cancer that added another layer of difficulty, "because it strips you of some of what makes you female."

Common sexual issues following cancer treatment for both men and women are decreased libido and other hormone-related issues. Women may also deal with vaginal issues, dryness, or discomfort during sex that can be brought on by "chemopause" or even actual menopause following treatment. For men, erections that aren't as firm or as frequent can be problematic. All of these issues can be heightened by depression, self-esteem, and body image concerns as well.

Dr. Bolte recommends getting to know your own body again before sharing it with someone else. "See what feels good to you, where the sensitivities are and what might trigger a negative experience. Listen to your body," she said.

Lynn, a prostate cancer survivor, said, "I function normally, but there is no ejaculation when I orgasm. It doesn't sound like a big deal, but for a guy, it kind of is. Sometimes I have pain too. Kind of like a knife stab when I orgasm." He said doctors don't know what causes the pain or what to do about it. "If you want to have a sexual relationship, you just deal with the pain," he said. Lynn also said he is not self-conscious about discussing these issues, not just with partners, but more widely. He, too, speaks about sexual issues post-cancer publicly to help other survivors.

Ethan Zohn, a 40-year-old former professional soccer player and reality-TV star, was diagnosed in 2009 with a rare type of Hodgkin's lymphoma. His treatment of intense chemotherapy and two stem cell transplants left him facing temporary sexual side effects as well. He makes light of it by comparing his dating life to that of Elaine from a famous *Seinfeld* episode. When her favorite form of birth control, the sponge, is discontinued, she has to ration her limited supply by deciding if her dates are "sponge-worthy."

When Ethan's insurance stopped covering Viagra or Cialis, he mentally added the $30 per pill cost onto his dates, and thought about the point in the evening when he had to determine what was coming next. "Do I pop the Viagra now? Is she Viagra-worthy?" he joked. "I didn't always know if I was reading the vibe the right way. Maybe it wouldn't even be necessary."

Though he laughs about it, he admits there was a serious side too. "I wasn't sure if I should tell them why I was taking Viagra," he says. "I didn't want them to feel insecure or think it had something to do with them." Navigating these kinds of situations can be tricky. "Do I ask her if this is going to the next level?" he wonders. "Do I want to take it to the next level? It puts a couple of layers of added complication on these kinds of situations that wasn't there before," he explains.

Another advocate who isn't shy about sharing is Jonny Imerman. For testicular cancer survivors, like him, the most difficult decision can be whether or not to get a prosthetic testicle. Jonny said those under 20 usually opt for the "fake ball," while older guys seem to not care about the aesthetics and balance issues involved, though they may choose a prosthetic because it's easier than disclosing their cancer. "Older guys usually realize women aren't concerned what your balls look or feel like," Jonny says. "As a result, they aren't as concerned about it either and usually opt out."

Collin, a 28-year-old testicular cancer survivor diagnosed at 21, says, "Don't get the fake ball." He did, and regrets it because he says it feels weird and doesn't hang right. People are intrigued by it, he said, but it wasn't necessary.

Jonny recommends seeking professional help if you are suffering from low self-esteem due to facial or other obvious scars, and in the case of sexual issues. There are experts who are trained to help you deal with these issues as well as survivors who are willing to talk openly about it and answer questions.

Dr. Bolte is one such expert. She has counseled hundreds of young adult survivors one-on-one and spoken before many more. She echoes Jonny's advice to seek professional help. Many cancer centers offer the services of a social worker or other counselors, and these professionals are trained to see more global issues than just psychological. They can provide a gateway to other types of assistance such as psychologists, psychiatrists, sex therapists, or other medical professionals if necessary.

Perhaps the best thing you can do for yourself immediately following cancer is to take the time you need to understand the new sexual you. It may not be the same as before, but that doesn't mean it has to be a struggle. There are many ways to experience pleasure sexually, and you may be called to be more inventive. The right partner will respect your needs and be willing to explore what works for both of you. And as Dr. Bolte says, your sexual health is important and valuable whether in a relationship or not.

What sexual issues have you dealt with before or after treatment?

Which sources of support are most appealing to you for sexual issues? Counseling, books, talking to other survivors, or something else?

What is most important to you in sexual relationships? What can you do to ensure your needs are met?

Marriage

A successful marriage requires falling in love many times,
always with the same person.
—Mignon McLaughlin

Don't marry the person you think you can live with; marry only
the individual you think you can't live without.
—James C. Dobson

In the two years I have been writing this book, several of the singles I interviewed aren't single anymore. Tamika and Jasan both got engaged and married during that time, while Leah and Heather Swift got engaged, the latter on stage at the Stupid Cancer OMG Conference in Las Vegas. It was quite exciting, and her fiancé Brian is very brave.

It turns out that marriage has positive effects for those diagnosed with cancer, at the same time that childhood cancer survivors experience less success with marriage according to some recent studies.

Survival rates increase by about 20 percent for married people according to a 2013 Harvard study. Men get the biggest benefits, and the study found that for breast and colon cancer patients, marriage benefits outweighed those from receiving chemo. Married people were more likely to catch cancer at an earlier stage, choose the right treatment, and stick with it, and they also had a 17 percent lower chance of their cancer spreading.

Researchers suggest that their findings don't necessarily proclaim any health benefits to marriage itself, but that social support plays a big role in the overall well-being of patients during a difficult time. They say that friends and loved ones can make a difference by going with the patient to doctor's appointments and treatments, and helping them understand their diagnosis.

A study from Great Britain with childhood cancer survivors showed that marriage rates were lower for adult survivors of childhood cancer, and that those who did marry had higher divorce rates than the general population, with men less likely to marry than women. Childhood cancer survivors were also more often found to be living with their parents.

For single men, these statistics are especially grim, as the research suggests they are generally not as good at marshaling support during difficult times as women are, which makes them less likely to successfully negotiate a difficult diagnosis.

Many of us are waiting longer to get married these days, and marriage rates in the United States have been declining steadily since 1960 when nearly 66 percent of women 15 and older were married. Today, that rate is only 50 percent. Some factors increase your chances of staying married once you do find the one. Income above $50,000 a year, religious affiliation of some kind, a college degree, parents who are still together, and getting married after the age of 25 all exert varying degrees of influence upon whether or not a marriage is successful.

(continued)

(*continued*)

> There is good news for marriage, though, as stability is improving. According to the book *For Better* by Tara Parker-Pope, about 23 percent of college graduates who married in the 1970s divorced within 10 years. For those who wed in the 1990s, the rate dropped to 16 percent. Research from the Wharton School in Pennsylvania shows that age at marriage is the single best predictor of success. Eighty-one-percent of college graduates who married after age 26 in the 1980s were still together 20 years later, while only 65 percent of those marrying before that age stayed hitched as long.

"I am now five years out and finally beginning to feel normal again," said a survivor who completed my survey of single survivors, "but in five years, I have not been on one date. I want to get married. I want a boyfriend. I just want to go on a date. But for now, I am a 42-year-old spinster who got breast cancer at age 37, lost her chance for children, and has yet to meet the man of my dreams."

For many of us, marriage has seemed like the brass ring (or gold ring, as the case may be) we have been striving for, but we all know that just getting married isn't the answer. Finding the right person to spend our lives with will ensure that we actually do have this person in our lives for the long haul. There is a fine line between settling and taking the risk to love someone who may not be perfect because, let's face it, no one is. I think taking the risk to love is worth it—even if it means overcoming the occasional heartbreak.

Fertility

The management of fertility is one of the most important functions of adulthood.
—GERMAINE GREER

She who was barren has borne seven children, but she who has had many sons pines away. The Lord brings death and makes alive; he brings down to the grave and raises up.
—THE BIBLE, SAMUEL 2:5

Though I never had a strong desire to have children, I used to worry about who would take care of me in my old age if I didn't. Then my friend reminded me that there is no guarantee that your children will look out for you, even if you have them. Marriage and family seems like a great protection against loneliness, but it isn't always, and that alone is not a great reason to seek them out.

Nearly all of the women I interviewed for this book and have met in my work have dealt with fertility issues of some kind. Men deal with this issue too, but for them, it is a simpler solution to bank sperm. In contrast, women have a higher success rate freezing embryos rather than just eggs, which adds another complicated layer to the equation.

Whether making a difficult decision about surgery that could impact fertility, or having concerns about the damage chemo can do to reproductive abilities, these are common issues faced by survivors. Trying for anyone, these issues can be more complicated when you are single. Not only do you have to make big decisions about your future on your own, but you also have to face the financial implications of freezing eggs or sperm or embryos, which is often not covered by insurance.

Survivors who participated in my survey shared the following about fertility issues:

> "On the rare occasions I have met men and we have gotten to the stage of talking about kids, I have been honest. They walk out and act as if something is wrong with me. I cannot find a man who appreciates me for me and accepts what I have been through just to be here today."

> "The docs gave me the option to freeze my sperm just in case, and I'm very glad I did because now it is looking like I'll be able to have kids."

> "I didn't have time to even think about it. Being stage III, I jumped into treatment. As a woman, it is much more complicated than for guys, and I think there should be more discussion and help."

> "Menopause is under control because of hormones, but with my eggs, thankfully, in a freezer, my sister will hopefully be able to carry a child for me."

"I would have liked to freeze my eggs once I received my diagnosis and before I began treatment. I wish insurance companies would cover most of that cost for women in this position."

———————————

"Six years after my last chemo and I still have quality of life issues. I became infertile, which was crushing because I really wanted to have children."

———————————

"My doctor didn't inform me about sterility until she absolutely knew it would affect me, which was almost too late. I had to convince her to let me take time to explore my options and was referred to a great clinic and introduced to Fertile Hope, which was great."(Fertile Hope provides reproductive health information, support, and hope to cancer patients whose medical treatments present the risk of infertility.)

———————————

"As a single woman in my late 30s who had tongue cancer twice, there is a tremendous amount of pressure to try to get pregnant, which I would have to do on my own, before my cancer returns again."

———————————

"It was hard going to a fertility specialist by myself and seeing all the couples trying to have a baby. I was so young. I didn't even know if I wanted kids, but I didn't want the option taken from me."

———————————

Michelle Whitlock writes beautifully in her memoir, *How I Lost My Uterus and Found My Voice*, about her fledgling romance and desire to have a family, and how both were complicated by a cervical cancer diagnosis at age 26. Like Tamika, Michelle speaks openly about the sexual dysfunction that often results from surgical treatment of cervical cancer. For Michelle, and many other women, having children was so important that it became a big part of her treatment plan. Making the decision to delay treatment in order to preserve fertility is becoming more common as patients are made more aware of the risks of infertility.

Nearly 65 percent of the single survivors surveyed said they were concerned about fertility issues. Luckily, there is a wealth of information and services to support survivors with these concerns (see the resources section for more). It is incredible how many people I know who have used some sort of fertility specialist or treatment—whether a survivor or not. One friend just had twins post-40 from both donor eggs and sperm, and carried the kiddos herself. Another used her own frozen eggs to conceive with donor sperm. A married couple in my sphere had their first child with in vitro fertilization (IVF) and then conceived twins naturally a few years later. Medical science is indeed a marvel, though it doesn't work for everyone. I also know women who have tried and failed to have kids of their own, and others who have successfully had families using surrogates or through adoption. Don't give up, and be sure you explore your options fully if having a family is important to you.

"Survivors are often concerned about fertility and whether parenting or having a child naturally is a priority," Dr. Bolte said. "There is a tremendous amount of loss and grief about this, whether partnered or single, and people need time to grieve that. There is so much emphasis on living strong, but we need to give ourselves permission to heal and grieve what we've lost while we learn to trust our bodies again."

She also suggests utilizing a support group so survivors recognize they aren't alone in what they are dealing with. Just hearing that others have the same struggles can be comforting. She said making sure support groups are professionally monitored is critical. Clinically licensed counselors, psychologists or psychiatrists, master's trained social workers, or other professionals are adequately trained to appropriately handle whatever arises.

Matt Zachary, founder of Stupid Cancer, felt fortunate to have been treated in a pediatric cancer ward for brain cancer in college because he said they do a good job of discussing future fertility concerns. He banked sperm at a cost of two grand a year, and after he was married discovered that he was actually still fertile, but barely, he said.

He and his wife tried for a year to conceive naturally, and eventually did IVF using fresh, not frozen, sperm. They found a great facility that touted an 80 percent success rate, and felt really lucky that their parents helped them pay for it. The costs associated can be astronomical.

Stupid Cancer is a nonprofit organization that empowers those affected by young adult cancer through innovative and award-winning programs and services. Young adults, a largely unknown group in the war on cancer, account for 72,000 new diagnoses each year. That's one every eight minutes. It's also seven times more than all pediatric cancers combined.

Alice was the one to bring up fertility with her doctors. "I was in the recovery room after my biopsy, and my friend asked if I was going to freeze my eggs," she said. "It was the first time I had considered the threat to my fertility. Thinking about this was the first time I really lost it about my diagnosis," she said. "I had always wanted to be a mom, and felt more connected to being a mom than being a wife."

She asked for a referral to a fertility clinic and was told to worry about it after surgery. "I had to press my doctor to be allowed to proceed with this process. I'm so glad I didn't wait. It can be complicated squeezing this in between surgery and chemo, especially when you are recovering. You could lose your window if you wait," Alice said. "I had to start immediately with hormone injections, and only had overnight to think about this."

"My boyfriend at the time said he wouldn't do this with me," Alice said. They were in the process of breaking up before her diagnosis, but he stuck around to help out and was still living with her. "My world was already so fragile and now it really dropped out the bottom. This was the shittiest moment of my entire cancer experience, and I felt very alone."

That terrible moment ended up being a huge gift, Alice said, because it led her to found Fertile Action, an advocacy organization for cancer survivors. The organization offers counseling and support and negotiates lower rates with fertility clinics and cryobanks. Alice is proud that she has been able to make this process easier and cheaper for other survivors.

Alice is now the glowing single mom of a newborn son, and Matt and his wife, Jessica, are the parents of four-year-old twins all as a result of in vitro fertilization.

Clinics that work with Fertile Action provide free initial consults (something Alice paid $500 for), provide their services at a deep discount for cancer survivors, and even offer compassionate care when patients just don't have the means at all. Fertility preservation is not mandated currently for insurance providers except in a few states, and only 20 percent of insurance plans offer any coverage for infertility treatments, according to Alice. Some medication is provided for breast and ovarian cancer survivors since the drugs are also prescribed as part of the treatment for many with these types of cancer. It remains to be seen how the Affordable Care Act will impact this issue.

How do you tell someone that you know wants kids (because he mentioned it in his online dating profile), that you probably won't be able to have them because you are now one ovary lighter and chemo poisoned your eggs? So many women spent much of their lives trying desperately not to get pregnant, and then, when the doctors tell you that you have the

Big C, one of the first issues they bring up, if you are lucky and have a good oncologist, is preserving fertility.

You can pay a bundle to freeze your eggs in hopes that someday Mr. Right will provide the sperm to create a new life, though freezing embryos nets you a better chance of success if you can find that sperm now. Lance Armstrong froze his swimmers when he was diagnosed, and was happy he did later when he and his wife decided they wanted a family. He was also surprised by the unexpected pregnancy of his girlfriend several years post-treatment and divorce, proving that doctors can't predict what might happen in the future.

I recognized early on that I never really wanted kids, and decided not to take any fertility preservation measures. For those who know they want at least the possibility of having a family, there are many avenues to consider.

How have you examined your own feelings about having a family? Do you know you want children, or are you following societal expectations in that regard?

How much are you willing to undergo to have a family? Financially? Emotionally? Physically?

Is having a child more important to you than having a partner? Would you do it on your own?

THREE

Living Beyond

7

You Are Inspirational

We shall draw from the heart of suffering
itself the means of inspiration and survival.
—WINSTON CHURCHILL

Inspiration comes to us slowly and quietly. . .
prime it with a little solitude.
—BRENDA UELAND

Inspiration takes many forms. You have likely been called inspirational because of the health challenges you've faced. Maybe having cancer has inspired you to do things you have always wanted to do, or given you the motivation to make significant changes in your life. This chapter will explore inspiration from a variety of angles, and it will share stories of single survivors who have used their own experience to transform themselves or to help others. You have already heard some of their stories in other parts of this book.

Challenges Are What Make Us Great

Growing up, my dad always shared his positive thinking pamphlets and tapes with me. There were so many invaluable lessons and messages in that material, and I remember one in particular about a girl who suffered serious injuries leading to partial paralysis. She went on to achieve some incredible things, and people said, "Imagine what she could have done if she hadn't been paralyzed." The speaker suggested instead that she achieved those things *because* she was paralyzed. His stance was that our challenges are what make us great.

It is the darkness and difficulty we face that reminds us how much we love the light. We need both in order to really grow. Booker T. Washington said, "Success is to be measured not so much by the position that one has reached in life as by the obstacles which he has overcome."

In just a cursory count, I come up with 14 single people I know, most of them survivors themselves, who have used their experience as inspiration to start something great that serves others. Would Sean Swarner have climbed Mount Everest and started Cancer Climber to help survivors live healthy, active lives if he hadn't had two childhood cancers; Would Brad Ludden have founded First Descents, giving young adult survivors outdoor adventure camps if his aunt hadn't been diagnosed; would Tonia Farman have started Athletes for Cancer, providing Hawaiian surf camps, among other adventures, if her brother hadn't died of leukemia? It seems unlikely.

Because of that terrible moment she described of facing her infertility, Alice founded Fertile Action to help other survivors with fertility concerns. Jonny shared why he started Imerman Angels after seeing others going through cancer alone. Tamika didn't want others to be uninformed as she was about the links between human papillomavirus (HPV) and cervical cancer, and Tamika & Friends was born. Rise Above It was started by Colin O'Donoghue to provide financial assistance for immediate needs to individuals and families dealing with cancer. After Colin's death, his brother Ryan and others kept the foundation going. I started Solo Survivors because I recognized how difficult it was to navigate a serious illness as a single person.

Countless others have written blogs or books, served as mentors, volunteered their time, and raised significant amounts of money for cancer-related charities and for research. Some have competed in triathlons, marathons, bike races, and other athletic endeavors they may not have even considered before. Cancer, like other challenges, offers us an opportunity to take a good hard look at our lives, and sometimes it inspires us to reach new heights we may not have seen before, much less aspired to.

What have you overcome in life that you are proud of?

How have your challenges made you great?

Is there anything you'd like to do for others?

An Inspiration to Others

in•spi•ra•tion [in-spuh-rey-shuhn] noun
A divine influence directly and immediately exerted upon the mind or soul.

It was almost entirely following my cancer diagnosis that people began to tell me that I was an inspiration to them. It made me extremely uncomfortable at first. It was difficult for me to accept those accolades because, from my point-of-view, I was just doing what needed to be done. I was living my life, day-by-day, waking up, getting dressed, going to work, and following my treatment plan. What was the alternative? To pull the covers up over my head and refuse to get out of bed?

Heather Swift agreed, saying, "People say, 'Oh you're so strong.' I think we all have this, and it comes out when we need it—when we're tested."

I finally came to accept that if people were inspired by me, I was in no position to deny them that. By deflecting their comments, I was invalidating their feelings and also ignoring my own value and worth. We have a difficult time accepting that which we don't feel we deserve, whether it be praise, gratitude, or love.

Many people have been inspired by my healthy diet to make changes of their own, and that is very gratifying to me. It is incredible to see the ripples those changes can make across the lives of people I come into contact with. I was inspired by those who came before me to find alternative cancer treatments through books and websites, and I am thrilled to be able to pass that information along to others.

In the past year, I was recognized by three different organizations for my work with hazing prevention. When I left my previous job of eight years following cancer treatment, I founded a nonprofit working mainly with colleges and universities to help them learn how to prevent this destructive and dangerous practice. It was very satisfying to receive these prestigious awards for work I was going to do anyway. I am grateful that my work in this area has inspired others to do more as well.

Krystal met Jonny Imerman when she was in the hospital. "I didn't want to continue the fight at that point," she said, "and Jonny connected me with someone else who had been fighting for three years and had had my surgery when it was in clinical trials. This gave me the courage to go for it." Because she was inspired by what Jonny was doing, she now works for Imerman Angels herself.

Marcia Donziger started MyLifeLine.org because of another survivor, Lori Andersen. The MLL website describes this impact: Marcia was profoundly inspired—not just by Lori's strength through crisis, but also by the way she harnessed the tools available to connect and communicate with her family and friends during her illness. Through Lori's own personal website, she posted her progress and courageously (and humorously!) inspired all who followed her struggle. As time went on, Lori's support network expanded beyond her imagination. People visited Lori's site to write encouraging messages, offer help to her family, or just stay updated and keep her in their prayers. Marcia saw the tremendous benefit for all families affected by cancer to communicate via a personal website. Through 2013, more than 116,000 people have registered on MyLifeLine.org to give or receive support from 175 countries and territories.

What a gift to be able to inspire someone else to find a new passion or strength within themselves. Most of the time, we never know how we may have inspired others, but you can bet that you have.

Has anyone ever told you that you are an inspiration to him or her?

How would you like to be inspiring to others?

Who inspires you? Why?

Try This
Who Inspires You?

Make a list of people who have inspired you. Can you list 5, 10, 20? Over the next month, work your way through the list, sending notes or making phone calls to each of the names on the list (add more as they come to you as well). Thank them for what they do and let them know how they have inspired you.

Live Life to the Fullest Every Day

Jenny, a cancer buddy I would likely never have met if mutual friends hadn't connected us due to a similar diagnosis, taught me about living life to the fullest. Though she had done chemo almost continuously for nearly three years, the cancer was winning, and she knew she would eventually die from the disease.

And yet she lived her life fully every day, spending time with friends and family, golfing, skiing, kayaking, and participating in other adventures that even 100 percent healthy people don't undertake. She traveled and spent quality time with her husband, and talked matter-of-factly about her future, or lack thereof. She was my idol in every way. I feel blessed to have met her, and learned from her.

I was connected to Alli Ward through Imerman Angels when I was assigned to be her mentor. I quickly realized I had nothing to teach this woman. Instead, she became an inspiration to me for the way she was handling her stage IV ovarian cancer diagnosis. She had so many great friends and tremendous support, but her body was ravaged by the disease and side effects from the drugs she was taking.

At first, Alli demurred when I talked to her about coming on a canoe trip I was organizing for single survivors. She didn't feel she was in good enough physical condition to handle paddling and camping for three days, though she missed doing the outdoor activities that had been a big part of her life before. I told her our small volunteer guide staff couldn't manage a trip with participants who were all in her condition, but one or two folks with physical challenges could be supported by the group. I felt really strongly that she needed to come.

In 2008, Alli's doctors gave her three to six months when her treatment didn't seem to be working. She had gone to this particular doctor appointment alone and, after the prognosis, made the decision to stop treatment on her own as well. She didn't want to spend her remaining time dealing with horrible side effects, so she stopped getting chemo, wrote good-bye letters to her friends and family, and got her affairs in order.

She would lie awake at night afraid that she was letting people down. Giving up. However, she was also relieved because she was tired of fighting, and wanted to enjoy her last days as much as possible. She never considered what she would do if she outlived her expiration date. She had cashed in her 401K, quit her job, sold her condo, and moved back in with her parents for support. She was experiencing constant nausea, seizures, abdominal and other pain, and she walked with the aid of a cane. The seizures kept her from driving, and she became even more dependent upon others.

On the canoe trip, Alli was often so sick that just making it through the day seemed like a tremendous effort. The group delivered meals to her perch in a comfy camp chair, and helped her out in numerous other ways. Sitting in the front of the canoe for several hours a day was difficult enough, let alone paddling.

"Luckily I had the best canoe partner, and all he asked from me was to tell him which side of the boat I would puke on so he didn't have to paddle through my vomit," Alli laughs. "I learned on that trip that you can feel like crap and still have fun. I think that was the start of a new beginning for me. I was no longer happy just sitting around in what had become a half-life. Terminal diagnosis or not, I was going to live."

Today, I hardly recognize Alli as the same woman who showed up for that canoe trip nearly four years ago (and two years after she was supposed to die). Even though the cancer has spread to her brain, and she is once again doing treatment, she has stopped using her cane, and having seizures, and has become physically active again. She has lost 40 pounds, is driving, and creates meaning in her life through her work at the Stupid Cancer Foundation.

In 2012, she embarked on a new adventure she dubbed Allipalooza. It involved whitewater kayaking with First Descents, traveling by van around the Southwest, participating in a 5K, dating, and visiting friends and family around the country. "I have been given a new chance to write the next chapter in my life," Alli says. "Recently someone asked me 'What happens if you get sick again?' My answer was simple 'What happens if I don't?'"

Try This
Life To Dos

What's on your bucket list? Do you already have one? When was the last time you reviewed it? Checked something off? Take it out and spend some time with it this week. Add items or cross off ones you've accomplished. If you don't already have one, start it today. What do you want to do, see, learn? Who would you like to meet? What books would you like to read? Where have you always dreamed of traveling to? If you're so inclined, share a few of your items on the Solo Survivors Facebook page #bucketlist so we can encourage each other in fulfilling our goals.

As I was sitting on a lanai in Kauai hours before my 40th birthday feeling a sense of accomplishment, peace, and gratitude, I thought of my friend Jenny. I have always had what I call a Life To Do List, and visiting all 50 states by the time I turned 40 was a long-time goal. When I was diagnosed with ovarian cancer, I had a handful of states left and meeting my goal became more of a priority. Six months before my 40th birthday only three remained: North Dakota, Oklahoma, and Hawaii.

Hawaii seemed like the perfect place to celebrate turning 40, so I booked a trip with a few friends over my birthday. I planned a camping and hiking trip over a long weekend in Theodore Roosevelt National Park and ticked North Dakota off of my list. Oklahoma proved more of a challenge. Two failed attempts due to weather and car problems had me sweating the deadline. I finally ended up flying to Oklahoma City for the day only a few days prior to leaving for Hawaii. On a bitterly cold January day, I visited the bombing memorial, had lunch at a great BBQ joint, and spent the afternoon at the Cowboy and Western Museum. My flight and rental car were birthday gifts from two different friends.

Some might feel depressed about turning 40, and the over-the-hill jests are a given as people liken this monumental milestone to the beginning of a downward spiral, but I know better. I have come closer than many my age to the alternative, and turning 40 was more than cause for celebration to me. I have not begun to reach the highest peaks of my life yet. Cancer helped me to realize this. And Jenny. And Alli. Their inspiration is ever-present. My dad always swore that life began at 40, and I believe him. I am coming into my own in my fourth decade of life, and I couldn't be happier.

How can you live your life more fully today?

What have you always wanted to do, learn, see?

What have you done post-cancer that you wouldn't have considered before?

An Opportunity for Transformation

A radical inner transformation and rise to a new level of consciousness might be the only real hope we have in the current global crisis brought on by the dominance of the Western mechanistic paradigm.
—STANISLAV GROF

People travel to wonder at the height of mountains, at the huge waves of the sea, at the long courses of rivers, at the vast compass of the ocean, at the circular motion of the stars; and they pass by themselves without wondering.
—ST. AUGUSTINE

We have all heard the analogy of the caterpillar turning into the butterfly as it fights its way out of the cocoon. It seems a bit cliché, but I honestly can't think of a better one to describe the past couple of years for me. I feel as if I've truly transformed from a crawling kind of creature (with some beauty to it for sure) into a flying, brilliant butterfly. While it might have been nice if something other than a cancer diagnosis had sparked this transformation, I am so grateful for the person I am now: lighter, more joyful, calmer in spirit.

If it hadn't been for cancer's wake up call, I might still be sleepwalking through life. I might not have ever realized how blessed I am, and how much I have to be thankful for. Cancer does wield some power over me, but it's the power to produce gratitude, to light a fire under me to get going on the things I want to do, and to connect me with other amazing people who have also been forged by this particular fire.

Krystal shared some significant transformations. "I have a different perspective and a new outlook on life after cancer," she said. Keeping her diagnosis mostly private throughout treatment, she said cancer taught her the importance of being open. "If it wasn't for someone being willing to share with me, I might not be here because I probably wouldn't have had the surgery. I have an obligation now to share my story if it will help other people."

"I believe things happen for a reason and God doesn't give you anything you can't handle," she says. "I used to worry about everything—money, jobs, decisions, etc. Little things. Now I live in the moment and realize that everything will work out and worrying about it doesn't help. I am a lot more laid back now, and willing to try new things, have fun, and enjoy my life."

I think a lot about transformation now, though I haven't found a definition in any dictionary that pinpoints exactly what I mean by it. For me, transformation is a lot about changing my perspective on life including:

How I show up in life—as I appear to others and from my own perspective

How I view situations—blame others or circumstances or take responsibility

How I relate to people—with distrust or giving them the benefit of the doubt

How I view the world—connected or separate

How I view myself—whole and complete or lacking in some way

What can you transform?

Your relationship with your parents?

Your relationship to money?

Your view of yourself?

Your view of Tea Partiers or terrorists or gay people?

What can you take responsibility for?

The fact that you have been playing the victim?

The way you react when someone pushes your buttons?

The way you spend money or eat when you are feeling depressed?

The way you hurt others when you are hurt?

What can you gain from seeing things differently?

Love instead of fear?

Tolerance instead of hate?

Joy instead of sadness?

Peace instead of conflict?

Once you have identified what you want to transform, you can work on developing a process similar to the one below that helps me feel centered and calm. (Based on teachings from *A Course in Miracles* and Landmark Education.)

1. I sit still somewhere and center myself with deep slow breaths.

2. Then I meditate or pray and simply ask to see it differently. Over and over if necessary. This doesn't usually come quickly.

3. Rather than placing blame, I look for something I can take responsibility for. Taking responsibility gives me the power to transform the experience.

4. Next, I look for the "story" I have been telling myself about the situation or about me or others involved. This is often based on past experience—"This always happens to me," "I am so stupid," "I'm not worthy of love," and so on. This can be a difficult step because our stories are our reality—they are the lens through which we view the world. They are such a part of us that they can be difficult to see. This is where an objective coach with some training might be helpful.

(continued)

(*continued*)

5. Be generous–what are the positives about this experience or person that I am currently struggling with? What opportunities is this experience opening up for me? How can my life be different as a result?

6. It helps me to journal or write a letter to the person or organization. Whether I send it or not, writing often helps me identify my own feelings so I can make sense of them.

7. Be authentic. This isn't about my ego or saving face or being right. It isn't about making the other person wrong. I write and work through these elements with I statements, to take ownership of my experiences in life. This process is so powerful to me that I am able to heal and move forward from challenging situations.

8. Finally, I let go of any attachment to the outcome, especially in relation to the other person. My request may go unfulfilled, and many times completely unheard. That doesn't matter. This is an internal exercise.

You can still forgive and let go even if the other party doesn't feel or show remorse, admit responsibility, or even receive the communication. This process is about transforming the experience for YOU alone.

From the day of diagnosis, Emily recognized that cancer could transform her life, and she asked it, "What are you here to teach me?" The answer she received was to slow down. Whoa! She described herself pre-cancer as a workaholic, and said that even though she had begun practices to help her be more peaceful, such as yoga and meditation, she was mostly just "going through the motions."

Even now as she is taking time away from work purposely to focus on allowing herself to completely heal, she said her inner chatter is always telling her: "You should be doing more, you aren't contributing enough unless you're working hard every day, and you're only loveable if you're producing something of importance."

"This egoic voice is always telling me I'm not enough, and not doing enough. It is what led me to work so hard and ignore my body's signs to take care of myself for so long. I believe cancer is just a big wake up call to take better care of ourselves," Emily says.

*What would you like to transform about the way you are living
your life?*

How would you live your life if you felt like you had permission to?

What has been transformational about cancer for you?

You Deserve a Guilt-Free Escape

*All the best stories are but one story in reality — the
story of escape. It is the only thing which interests us all,
and at all times, how to escape.*
—A.C. BENSON

*If you are patient in one moment of anger, you will escape one
hundred days of sorrow.*
—CHINESE PROVERB

When you are going through something difficult, like cancer, it is important to find a way to take some time for yourself without guilt. As Emily shared, her time for herself won't do much good if she spends all of it feeling that she should be doing something else. Don't think about what you should be doing instead. Don't worry what other people think. Find a healthy escape that works for you whether it's for 15 minutes, a few hours, a week, or even more.

Finding healthy escapes became a priority for me after my cancer diagnosis. My chiropractor surprised me one day by asking me to repeat the phrase, "I am a good person and I deserve some time for myself." The first time I tried to say it, I couldn't. I was too choked up. How had he recognized my guilt at taking time for me, when I hadn't seen it? He had me say this over and over again until I could do it easily.

My ideal escape is experiencing nature for long stretches of time. As a whitewater canoe guide, these trips have always fed my soul, but one week-long trip on the Green River in Utah with friends was magical. It comes up over and over again when this group of friends gets together. We tell the stories, remember the beauty and peace and fellowship we experienced around the campfire at night, and in some way recreate the feelings as well. This trip continued to pay dividends long after the canoes were loaded back onto the trailer for the long drive home.

It is great to take a week or two away to relax and really unwind, but when that's not possible, mini-escapes can be good as well: yoga, a walk, reading a book, writing, talking to a friend, or meditating. Even a nap can feel like an amazing gift to ourselves. Though we resisted them as young children, naps now seem like such luxurious treats.

The best escapes are those that feed your body or mind (or both!). It's easy to use television, food, alcohol, or drugs as an escape, and while those may provide momentary relief from fear, pain, or other difficult emotions, they won't provide lasting benefits—the opposite, in fact. Did you know that watching four hours of television a day equates to 13 years over the average lifespan?

That's 13 years watching other people, usually fictional people, do amazing, stupid, crazy, and often destructive things. Studies have shown that people who watch a lot of television have a more negative view of the world because we equate the murder and mayhem we see on television with reality. Even though I still watch more television than I would like, I'm so much more aware now of how precious my time is. Even when I need to escape from my life for a bit, I want to use the time on something that fulfills me.

Try This

Great Escapes

How do you escape? List the ways you leave your life behind. Take a careful look at your list. Do these escapes rejuvenate, motivate, or sustain you? Or do they numb, sadden, or cause regret? (Hint: One way to tell is to think about how you feel at the end of them. Imagine yourself after a night of heavy drinking, and after a long dinner with a friend.) Place a star next to the ones in the first category. How can you bring more healthy escapes into your life? Who might be able to help you do so?

Healthy escapes can renew you in a way that a pull-the-covers-over-your-head kind of escape usually doesn't. No matter what you do, once you've done it, don't beat yourself up about anything that you judge you "shouldn't have done." Just recognize that it didn't serve you, and in the future you can remember that feeling to help you choose something healthier for your body and soul.

We sometimes feel guilty about escaping, feeling that we should be doing something else instead. What is so interesting about inspiration, though, is that it often strikes when you least expect it. Trying to solve a difficult problem at work? Sometimes a walk around the block will provide an idea more quickly than sitting at your desk reviewing data. Getting out of our own heads, even if just for a short time, often brings out creativity in unexpected ways.

Yes, there are times when we need to buckle down and focus on a project, and there are others when allowing, rather than trying to force, new ideas is a better approach. There is a reason many tech companies offer pingpong tables, volleyball courts, and other creative work spaces for people to collaborate. Innovative thinking comes from this type of environment. You can create your own kind of inspirational environment in your home or office, and remember the power of escape to sometimes allow those great ideas to bubble to the surface.

What would be your perfect escape?

How can you make it happen?

When time is an issue, which parts of your ideal escape can you sneak into your day?

Which circumstances have brought ideas when you least expected them?

8

You Are Powerful

Our deepest fear is not that we are inadequate.
Our deepest fear is that we are powerful beyond measure.
It is our Light, not our Darkness, that most frightens us.
—MARIANNE WILLIAMSON

He who controls others may be powerful, but he who
has mastered himself is mightier still.
—LAO TZU

We are powerful, and sometimes that scares us. The term "power" has gotten a bad rap. Often equated with greed, social climbing, and even taking advantage of others, we can see powerful people as puppet-masters pulling the strings of society, and doing so in a way that primarily benefits themselves and their kind.

With that view, being powerful doesn't always seem so appealing. Instead, owning our power involves taking responsibility for our own lives and recognizing the impact our actions have on others and ourselves. When we own our power, we interact with people differently, not sharing complaints and problems and blaming each other for them, but relating in a way that is affirming and peaceful instead. Owning our power doesn't allow us to play victim.

Four years after my initial diagnosis, and just a few weeks prior to my first recurrence, 14 single survivors from across the country joined me for a three-day adventure on the Colorado River. Since I had been talking about providing services for the single survivor crowd for a long time, that trip was a big deal for me. Turns out, it was a big deal for them too. The trip was so rewarding and fun for us all, and significantly life-changing for a few. Two of the participants dated each other for several months following the trip, and others gained a new perspective that has altered the direction of their lives. Here are just a few of the comments from the weekend:

"Thanks for four of the best days of my life. It's been a LONG time since I've felt joy and at peace, and this weekend I felt both. Also, I feel hopeful again, and inspired to get out there and really live. Thank you SOOO much!"

—*Alli Ward*

"I just wanted to say thank you for this weekend. It was something I really needed and came at the right time. I'm sure everyone on the trip had the best time of their lives, and you touched more lives than you can imagine—not just those attending, but those who are their friends, their family. . .etc. It's quite amazing to see the change in people and you were the catalyst for that change. It was an honor to be a part of this event and I can't thank you enough."

—*Sean Swarner*

When I started planning the trip, I could never have imagined the profound impact it would have on some of the participants, and on me. To know that I could do work that would contribute so strongly to people's sense of themselves, and provide them with hope for the future, was astounding. It was after that trip that I began to really acknowledge my own power, and see what I could do when I, myself, stopped playing small and really went for it. I will never take for granted again the power that I have to make a difference.

The Power of Gratitude

Develop an attitude of gratitude, and give thanks for everything that happens to you, knowing that every step forward is a step toward achieving something bigger and better than your current situation.
—BRIAN TRACY

Gratitude unlocks the fullness of life. It turns what we have into enough, and more. It turns denial into acceptance, chaos to order, confusion to clarity. It can turn a meal into a feast, a house into a home, a stranger into a friend.
—MELODY BEATTIE

It is so easy to get wrapped up in what is missing from our lives. The lack of boyfriend, fulfilling job, or fat paycheck can loom large in our thoughts, causing us frustration and disappointment. We tell ourselves that we need certain things to be happy, which only makes us "needy." Our thoughts then become a self-fulfilling prophecy, ensuring that our focus on what's lacking will create more of the same. These negative thoughts, such as, "I will always be alone," "I'm not good enough," "I'm too fat," contribute to a deep feeling of disempowerment that will keep us from getting what we want.

Focusing on and appreciating what we have is the best way to create more good things in our lives. Let's face it, just by virtue of living in a first-world country, we have it better than most people in the world. Access to clean water, healthy food, and medical care are givens in most of our lives. We are surrounded by abundance and comfort, and don't always appreciate just how good we have it.

Over the years, I have often complained about "being alone." In between boyfriends or during a dry dating spell, as friends around me got married and started families, I felt sorry for myself for what was missing. The loneliness, and sometimes even despair, was so palpable in my life that it blinded me to all the good things. Even when I was visiting somewhere amazing, as I often do, I would be sad that I didn't have someone to share it with.

The truth is that I have never been alone. I could literally drown in the sea of love in which I have been fortunate enough to swim my entire life. Getting cancer was a fantastic reminder of just how many people care about me. I was overwhelmed by the outpouring of love and support from friends, family, coworkers, people I hadn't seen or been in touch with for years, friends of friends, religious communities, and cancer-related organizations, just to name a few. I received tons of notes and cards, not to mention all the flowers, gifts, meals, and visits, and the people in my life raised nearly $10,000 for ovarian cancer research in my honor.

I am astounded that I could be in the midst of all of that and still feel alone in any way, shape, or form. I may live alone in a one-bedroom condo, work from home without colleagues around, and file my taxes as a single person, but I am FAR from alone! I am truly and deeply loved by so many people. If you take stock of your life, you will realize that you are too.

Sometimes it takes something "bad," such as an illness or injury, to help us realize all the "good" in our lives.

Often when we are going through a difficult time, people remind us that it could be much worse. I just did that with my previous first-world comment above. While sometimes this helps us put things into perspective, other times it makes us feel like ungrateful wretches. Ingratitude isn't a weapon you should use to bludgeon yourself. It's important not to resist whatever you're feeling. Whatever you feel is fine. Acknowledge and honor your feelings, while also recognizing that wallowing in them forever won't serve you.

I am profoundly grateful for the love of my family and so many friends, and I love my life so much. I know that it will be enhanced when I find a partner to share it with, but it's pretty freaking amazing right now. On a trip to Maui, I drove to the top of the volcanic crater to watch the sunrise one morning, and found myself surrounded by honeymooning couples and families of all kinds. I was the only one there on my own. I began to feel sorry for myself, and then I remembered that I could act "as if," and I conjured up feelings of what it would be like to share that incredible view with someone special. I also thought about all the other places I could be at that moment, and realized how blessed I was to be sitting on top of the world, watching the sunrise. Instantly, I felt differently.

I often feel lonely, and wish I had a partner to share those special moments with, but I know that feeling what it will be like to share my life with an amazing man will actually attract that special someone to me. Visualizations are powerful tools to transforming whatever experience we are having into something better, and the bonus is that doing them often enough can attract what we want as well. Instead of saying "I'll believe it when I see it," Zig Ziglar reminded us, "I will see it when I believe it."

Try This

Gratitude Practice

If you're not into keeping a gratitude journal, find another way to express your daily gratitude—a morning or evening meditation, a blessing when walking out of or into the front door for what you're going to do or coming home to, or whatever works for you.

What in your life are you grateful for?

The Fire of Commitment

*There's a difference between interest and commitment.
When you're interested in doing something, you do it only when
circumstances permit. When you're committed to something,
you accept no excuses, only results.*
—ART TUROCK

*It was character that got us out of bed, commitment
that moved us into action and discipline that
enabled us to follow through.*
—ZIG ZIGLAR

I loved Elizabeth Gilbert's book *Committed*. It is about the history of marriage, her disdain for it as a concept, and her eventual surrender to it. My sisters are both married, and one of them told me once that she could feel secure through the rough times in her marriage—the disagreements and arguments and tensions—because she knew her husband wasn't going anywhere. They were committed, and therefore safe to share their true feelings, allow themselves to be vulnerable, and assert their perspective. As a single person, that resonated so deeply with me, and confirmed my willingness to wait for that kind of relationship as well.

Commitment might seem like a strange topic for a book about single life, but commitment is important in all areas of life, not just romantic relationships. This quote by W. H. Murray of the Scottish Himalayan Expedition sums it up:

> Until one is committed, there is hesitancy, the chance to draw back, always ineffectiveness. Concerning all acts of initiative and creation, there is one elementary truth the ignorance of which kills countless ideas and splendid plans: that the moment one definitely commits oneself, then providence moves too. All sorts of things occur to help one that would never otherwise have occurred. A whole stream of events issues from the decision, raising in one's favor all manner of unforeseen incidents, meetings, and material assistance which no man could have dreamed would have come his way. I have learned a deep respect for one of Goethe's couplets: "Whatever you can do, or dream you can, begin it! Boldness has genius, magic, and power in it."

This book came about because I made a commitment to it. I set an intention, and began taking actions in that direction. For five years I had been talking about writing a book, and hoping to be discovered though my blog, but it wasn't until I made a commitment and took action that it actually happened. I joined a group of other women who wanted to write books, reading *How to Bring Your Book to Life This Year*. I attended an author conference in Las Vegas with a friend. This event was rife with publishers, agents, marketing gurus, book designers, and others. I made great connections, learned a ton about the publishing industry, and, most importantly, began to see myself as an author and speaker with a message that can make a difference to people.

I came home and started putting together a press kit, surprising myself at how many media interviews I had done over the past few years on this topic. I stayed up late to work on this one night, and the very next day, the publisher of this book sent me an e-mail to let me know she thought the subject of my blog would make a great book. Coincidence? Absolutely not!

Try This

The Fire of Commitment

Take a moment to explore and write down the things you are committed to today. It is only through setting the intention and/ or making the commitment that they will come to you. Once you've set an intention, let go of any fixation on the way it might come to fruition.

For example, I am committed to:

- Living an adventurous life
- Enjoying complete freedom over my schedule (doing what I want, when I want)
- Making a contribution in the world through my words and actions
- Generating abundance in the form of love, prosperity, peace, and joy
- Finding a life partner who loves and supports me

In the Unitarian Universalist church, we light a chalice at the beginning of each service, and at the end, when we extinguish it, we say the following: "We extinguish this flame, but not the light of truth, the warmth of community, or the fire of commitment. These we carry in our hearts until we are together again." I wish for you the fire of commitment.

What are YOU committed to?

What actions will you take right now to achieve what you're committed to?

Who can you engage to help you AND hold you accountable for those actions?

The Power of Possibility

> *There is one consolation in being sick; and that is the possibility that you may recover to a better state than you were ever in before.*
> —HENRY DAVID THOREAU

> *Trust yourself. Create the kind of self that you will be happy to live with all your life. Make the most of yourself by fanning the tiny, inner sparks of possibility into flames of achievement.*
> —GOLDA MEIR

Possibility is a beautiful word. It is hope and potential and believing in what could be. It is the basis of quantum physics (in the very simplest terms), which suggests that the mere act of observing something impacts its outcome. In other words, we create our world through the possibilities we perceive, and bring those possibilities to fruition through the power of those perceptions. There is no such thing as how the world is. There is only how we see the world.

I have been engaged for some time in programs through Landmark Education that have opened me up to living life in possibility. They suggest you can have anything you want for yourself and your life through creating a possibility and enrolling others in that possibility. This entails living without pressure, expectation, or attachment to any particular outcome inside of the possibility you have created, whether it be love, abundance, peace, or something else.

It means practicing living life powerfully, and living a life that I love. There is so much I have learned and practiced in this education, but perhaps most powerful is the concept of declaring an intention, or possibility, and then living into it as my word. Meaning that because I have given my word to it, I will consciously live in the space of that possibility, whatever it is.

I've made power a possibility, and I have been absolutely astounded at how much power has shown up for me in recent years. Power over my emotions, thoughts, actions; power to make a difference in the world; power to create what I desire; and owning the power of who I am rather than playing small.

I've learned the most about the benefits of living a life of possibility through the very first possibility I created: love. I had been insisting for months that a certain guy would eventually fall in love with me while he spent the same several months insisting he wouldn't. We were both miserable and at a complete standstill. Our friendship suffered, something neither of us wanted. Only after we were both able to open up to each other about our relationship baggage and our fears were we able to choose to explore what else might be possible for us together.

Almost as soon as we declared an openness to the possibility without the expectation of a specific outcome, everything changed for us. A weight was lifted. He stopped insisting he wouldn't fall in love with me, and I stopped insisting that I would fall in love with him. Our conversations became lighter and more open. We began to marvel in the relationship we do have, and enjoy it for what it is, without being attached to how or when or what that might look like. And indeed, we began saying, "I love you" to each other regularly.

Try This
Thoughts Become Things

I've found this practice based on work by Mike Dooley, author of *Leveraging the Universe*, helpful in bringing my dreams to life.

1. Set an intention, and give it to the universe. Don't worry about HOW it will come to pass; let the universe find the most efficient and effective path for your intention. By fixating on a certain path, we limit other opportunities that might not even be on our radar.

2. Be open to opportunities that could help manifest your intention, and take action. You don't have to see how each step will lead to your desired outcome all at once. Just take one step at a time. What is there to do right now? Who could you call? What could you learn?

3. NOTE: Intentions can look very different from goals, which are often time-based and specific, and different still from

possibilities. I have included examples of all three below
to clarify. No matter which one you use (or a combination
of all of them), they will lead you toward actions to take in
order to fulfill them.

Goal:
To have a million dollars in the bank by December 31, 2017.
Intention:
To have the freedom to do what I want, when I want.
Possibility:
Abundance and Generosity

What possibilities would you like to "live into?"

What intentions do you have for your life?

What goals are important to you?

The Power of Surrender

> *If you surrender completely to the moments as they*
> *pass, you live more richly those moments.*
> —ANNE MORROW LINDBERGH

> *To be able to love and live in freedom means to be able to*
> *make godly decisions. To make godly decisions we have to surrender our*
> *egos and all the falsity and shame that goes with it.*
> —JAMES MCGREEVEY

Surrender can feel significantly like defeat. We are always told to never surrender, never give up, never quit. To most of us, the idea of surrender is not only
negative, but actually shameful. We feel the need to stick it out, suck it up,
walk it off, and keep calm and carry on, no matter what! Surrendering equates
with losing, giving something away, or getting the short end of the stick.

I would like to suggest that the opposite is actually true. Surrender can
be powerful. It can provide peace. Have you ever heard the phrase, "What
you resist, persists?" We often resist that which we see as painful or shameful.
If we don't see it, don't feel it, and deny its existence, it will disappear, right?
Um. . .probably not. Resisting something puts all your attention on the thing

you are resisting. It gives energy to that which you want to avoid. What we focus on, expands.

Two recent situations have helped me see the benefit of surrendering my need for control and relinquishing my vision of how something would play out. One involved work and the other a personal relationship. Both were extremely challenging to me over an extended period of time, and I'm sure caused no end of angst for the other people involved as well. But once I made the decision to surrender, I felt lighter, more at ease, and freer. Though the "rightness" of my stance occasionally reared its ugly head during both processes, I also felt freedom when I could let it go. Releasing my need for control, I also let go of the weight of responsibility for making things work out, and could rest easy that other hands were carrying some of the burden.

Give some thought to the things you could surrender to. Not surrender, but surrender to. As in, not having to control every little aspect of everything in your life. I like to think of it this way: I have cancer, but it doesn't have me. I can give up my need for a particular outcome or test result in order to feel calm about my situation. I recognize that my worrying about it and trying desperately to control it won't necessarily make a difference, but surrendering can give me peace of mind without impacting my health. Or it might even have a positive effect as I am no longer stressed constantly about what might be going on in there.

About a decade ago, Laura Doyle ignited a firestorm with her *Surrendered* books for wives and singles, suggesting that women surrender to their men and stop trying to control the way the relationship was going. She advised respecting men's decisions for their lives, practicing good self-care, expressing gratitude for the things others do for you, and allowing yourself to be vulnerable.

The idea of surrendering stirred up controversy among some who hadn't read the books and who misinterpreted the premise to be about submission to men's desires and needs at the expense of our own (something perhaps women tend toward already). One human rights activist even went so far as to liken this approach to slavery, suggesting that the author expected women to subvert themselves entirely to their man, becoming a kind of puppet.

I remember the hubbub around the books when they came out, and admit to feeling a significant amount of distaste for the idea of surrender, even buying into the feminist outrage about the misrepresentation of this concept. I had no interest in reading the book then—why would I want to surrender my control?

I am absolutely intrigued by this idea now, loved the book, and totally see the power of surrender. It goes beyond gender issues, and speaks only of letting go and knowing that I don't have to try to steer the outcome of every single thing in my life. Whew! What an incredible feeling to trust other people to take care of it, trust the process to produce a great result, or even, as my intuition whispered to me recently, trust love, and know that whatever form it takes, it is real and I don't have to manipulate it in any way.

I want to clarify that I'm not suggesting you live your life at the whim of others, exerting no control over it. Only that you recognize that many of the things we try to control are things upon which we don't actually have any influence, such as how someone else feels about us, or how certain events will play out. Giving up the feeling that we have to try to control it can release a tremendous amount of stress.

Even though there are sure to be moments that scream for me to wield some sort of influence, assert my opinion, or just feel strongly that something must be WRONG, surrendering, in and of itself, is nothing short of blissful. I recognize there are numerous routes that lead to the same end, and that the view from the passenger seat can be really great and quite relaxing. The destination itself may even look different than expected, and that is OK too.

What are you trying to control that is stressing you out?

What would surrender create in this situation?

What would it look like to surrender to these experiences?

The Power to Heal

*Healing is a matter of time, but it is
sometimes also a matter of opportunity.*
—HIPPOCRATES *(460 BC–370 BC)*

*On the path to wellness one must learn to
recognize fear. Particularly within ourselves.
Anger is fear, jealousy is fear, even some ignorance.
Health, however, is born from love.*
—ANONYMOUS

For a year and a half, I walked around with the awareness of first two, and then six, masses growing in my body. All the tests and scans showed that they were actually growing, though not enough to cause me any problems for a long time. I had no symptoms, and I often forgot those little buggers were there. When people asked me about my health, I typically responded that I was fine before I remembered that, actually, there was something going on.

I believed my body could either live with those masses or expel them when needed. The fact that they were there, surprisingly, didn't bother me. They must be here to teach me something, I thought, and perhaps when I learn the lesson, they will no longer be needed. I was at peace about the situation, and that was powerful. I was so grateful not to be wracked with worry and fear every time something new happened regarding my health. It reminded me that it is possible to be peaceful in the face of any reality.

Viktor Frankl's book *Man's Search for Meaning* details his experiences in a Nazi concentration camp. Throughout his entire ordeal, and all the suffering and death he witnessed all around him, he focused on what he had to live for, thought about his wife and family, and helped others around him with his skills as a neurologist and psychiatrist. His attitude was that his captors could control his body, but they couldn't affect his mind. His outward circumstances had little impact on his internal state. In a place where only 1 in 28 prisoners survived the camps, Frankl's story is incredible. First published in 1946, his books about the philosophy that kept him alive have sold millions of copies, and he lived to be 92.

Dr. Frankl said it best, "We must never forget that we may also find meaning in life even when confronted with a hopeless situation, when facing a fate that cannot be changed. For what then matters is to bear witness to the uniquely human potential at its best, which is to transform a personal tragedy into a triumph, to turn one's predicament into a human achievement. When we are no longer able to change a situation—just think of an incurable disease such as inoperable cancer—we are challenged to change ourselves."

Not only can we control how we feel about it, many believe we can actually heal ourselves just with the power of our beliefs. We have long accepted the existence of the placebo effect—the idea that giving patients saline injections or sugar pills (with no active drug agents) will make them better, simply because they believe it will. They believe in the expertise of their doctor, and the efficacy of the "drug" they are being given. The placebo effect is controlled for in scientific studies, and has been demonstrated time and again to account for a fairly significant number of cures in clinical trials.

As the daughter of a physician and an MD herself, Rankin was skeptical about the idea that people could self-heal. She had been taught to believe only in that which could be measured, so she went in search of scientific proof of our ability to heal ourselves. Her book *Mind Over Medicine* presents that evidence, citing scientific studies published in peer-reviewed medical journals. She also shares cases from the Spontaneous Remission Project, a bibliography detailing the disappearance of disease without medical treatment.

Rankin shares one particularly powerful story in both her TED Talk and her book about a terminal cancer patient in 1957. All the treatments had failed, and with numerous large tumors throughout his body he was given only a week to live. The patient found out about a new drug being offered in clinical trials, and begged his doctor to put him on it. The patient didn't qualify for the trial that was limited to those believed to have at least three months left, but the doctor provided the drug anyway, giving the injection on a Friday afternoon, but not expecting to see his patient alive the following week. On Monday morning, the doctor was shocked to find the patient out of bed and walking around. Tests showed the tumors had shrunk in half, and 10 days after the first dose, the patient left the hospital.

For two months, the patient thrived, until medical journals began to report that this particular drug wasn't as effective as originally believed. The patient believed the reports, despite his own evidence to the contrary; he fell into a deep depression and the cancer returned. His doctor saw what happened and suspected the placebo effect at work, so he called the patient into his office and told him that some of the drug had been contaminated, resulting in the poor trial results. He had gotten a pure form of the drug and wanted to put the patient back on it.

The doctor injected the patient with distilled water, and again, the tumors in his chest dissipated, and the patient thrived for another two months. When the American Medical Association reported widely that the drug was a dismal failure, the patient lost faith in his treatment. The tumors returned and the patient died in two days.

I have struggled with these concepts. While I truly do believe that we have the power to heal ourselves, I have also been frustrated that I haven't been able to do it—*yet*. Despite my healthy diet, meditation, energy work, and natural cancer therapies, the cancer keeps coming back, and no matter how many times we remove the tumors, they have so far continued to return. It would be easy for me to believe nothing I am doing is working, and succumb to frustration and despair. Is my faith not strong enough? Are my thoughts not pure enough? What am I doing wrong?

Then I remember all of the things I am sharing with you. I am enough. I am doing the best I can with what I know now. I am actually feeling great, so why worry? I remember surrender. I remember to focus on the best case scenario. I remember to embrace my own power. I don't fall into despair only because I truly do look at all of life's challenges as opportunities to learn something. Being single, dealing with cancer, and struggling financially are all great teachers. They allow me to practice NOT making myself wrong. They require me to have faith that everything will be OK.

There is a great quote from the movie *The Best Exotic Marigold Hotel* that sums this up beautifully. The hotel manager says, "Everything will be alright in the end. . .if it's not alright, it's not yet the end." When I embrace this philosophy and remember the adorable Indian accent in which it was delivered, I can't help but smile while being reminded that this too shall pass, and I get to choose how I feel right now. And right now. And right now. And so do you.

What do you know when it comes to your own power to heal?

What could you surrender to right now?

The Power of Faith

Faith is knowledge within the heart,
beyond the reach of proof.
—KHALIL GIBRAN

Faith is taking the first step even when
you don't see the whole staircase.
—MARTIN LUTHER KING, JR.

There are volumes that could be written about this topic, in fact, they have been. I am only touching on it in a very brief and cursory way through sharing a bit of my own perspective as well as some other single survivors, including the most powerful story of a faith healing that has ever happened to someone I know personally.

I grew up in the Bible belt in a family that wasn't religious. Setting aside the inherent difficulties in that, I always associated faith with religion, and didn't think it had much of a place in my life. I rejected organized religion for a long time, and I realized after finding a church that resonated strongly with my beliefs that, during that time, I had also thrown God out with the bathwater. Though I still don't consider myself particularly religious, I am deeply spiritual, and becoming more so each day. I recently began to focus much more on the role of faith in my life, and to really trust in something bigger than myself more fervently than I have before.

Though I have always been a positive and hopeful person, there was a sort of block when it came to faith. I wanted evidence before I could trust. I believed that science and faith were at odds with each other, and that faith required a suspension of reason. I wanted to believe some of the things I was reading and hearing about the nature of the universe and the metaphysical, but I was skeptical and sometimes even cynical.

I now see that faith and science are actually intertwined, and there have been a number of scientific studies that have proven the healing power of faith and prayer. Conjuring up images of the miracles of Jesus, and the more modern evangelical tent revival healings, this is a difficult concept for many of us to accept.

And in addition to providing examples of the placebo effect, Rankin's book also discusses the nocebo effect, in which dire predictions by doctors and others can actually bring about those results. In one example, a midwife who delivered triplets on Friday the 13th said they were cursed and predicted each of their deaths at different ages. Each one dutifully died as foretold, two of them the day before the fateful birthday, the last with no discernible illness or cause of death after having checked herself into a hospital because of her fear, and having witnessed the fate of both sisters.

Quantum physics is gaining traction as an explanation of how our thoughts affect our physical surroundings and circumstances. Masaru Emoto demonstrated that human consciousness has an effect on the molecular structure of water. His experiments involved exposing water samples to concentrated thoughts of either a positive or a negative nature. Thoughts such as "you make me sick," "I hate you," and so on, were juxtaposed with loving and positive thoughts. Water frozen and examined under a microscope showed incomplete, malformed, and distorted crystals from the negative thoughts and beautiful, symmetrical, colorful patterns from the positive ones.

Even one of the most brilliant and famous scientists of all time, Albert Einstein, shared a definition of the divine that is similar to my own: "That deep emotional conviction of the presence of a superior reasoning power, which is revealed in the incomprehensible universe, forms my idea of God."

I participated in a program for young adult cancer survivors in Hawaii one spring. This surf camp asked us to choose a camp name that represented our power, and I chose Kale'le', which means "to have faith" in Hawaiian. I chose this, not because I already had an abundance of faith, but because I was seeking to foster more of it in my life. I awaken each day to a sign above my bed that reads, "I trust that I will be taken care of." And I really do. Since I have been practicing a higher level of faith in my life, I have been able to remain peaceful despite uncertain health and inconsistent income.

In the past, I worried a great deal. I didn't necessarily express my worries to others, but internally, I was always focused on what was "wrong," and on the problems in my life. Now, I choose to focus on the positives and the possibilities instead. It's a subtle shift with profound implications. The circumstances of my life haven't changed dramatically, but my inner state about them has. I am much calmer, more peaceful, grateful, and loving in my thoughts.

In the past, I often viewed religion as a sort of crutch, giving the faithful a certainty that was comforting, no doubt, but providing little basis in reality. Sure, it was helpful in getting through day-to-day life, but wasn't it also folly of a sort to believe in something for which there was no evidence? Now I see that there is no downside to faith. If we believe in something bigger than ourselves and are wrong, we've lost nothing, but if that belief gives us comfort in life, we've gained a great deal.

Emily Hine was diagnosed with stage II uterine cancer at age 44, and from the very start, she received spiritual signs not to have surgery or radiation. At that time, she had already been following signs about her personal and professional life for a few years and producing some magical results, but could she really do it with her health as well, she wondered?

She found a doctor who shared her point of view and "spoke her language," as she describes it. She went on a natural regimen of supplements prescribed by this physician and began a nutritional detox program. She said the most difficult part was overcoming the fears and doubts of her friends and family about her approach.

Emily said, "I realized that I needed to take action to do my part in the healing process. That included finding the right health care team, having a back-up plan that included surgery as a last resort, detoxing, and eating healthier. When I did my part, spirit came in with a miraculous 'spiritual surgery' that wasn't precipitated by any treatment."

Because this experience occurred as a lucid dream, Emily said she herself might have ignored it if it hadn't come with physical evidence afterward. "I had a hard time believing it really happened," Emily said. "The evidence was comforting." She details her entire healing experience in her blog, Holy Sit. "I do think what's important and will serve others is a multi-pronged approach: western medicine, alternative therapies, and a belief that you are already well," Emily said.

What does having faith mean to you?

What connects you to the idea of something bigger than yourself?

How has your faith or trust served you in life and in dealing with cancer?

9

You Are Loved

*Being deeply loved by someone gives you strength,
while loving someone deeply gives you courage.*
—*Lao Tzu*

*A loving person lives in a loving world. A hostile person lives in a
hostile world. Every person you meet is your mirror.*
—*Ken Keyes*

"Love is the answer." We hear it all the time. In song lyrics, poems, books, and movies. Love is the key to everything. It is the be all, end all. The only thing that matters. I believe this sentiment is true. That love is the cure for what ails us, literally and figuratively.

Often, it feels as if love is the only thing missing from my life, but only when I subscribe to a very narrow definition of love—one that includes only romantic or soul-mate love. One that leaves out agape (charity or compassion), philia (friendship), parental love, love of the divine (spiritual), brotherly love (love for your fellow man), eros (passionate or sexual love), and self-love. We all enjoy one or many of these types of love in our lives. And yet we often feel the void of love if we aren't "in love" with someone special, or if we are in love with someone who doesn't return our affection. We turn our backs on the numerous other types of love that are always present. We confer on them lesser-than status.

Because I was tired of focusing on what was missing from my life in the form of romantic love, I began to explore love in its many forms, the importance of love in health, and ways I could appreciate the love I have. I then sought to cultivate more of it in my life, including the elusive self-love, which is so crucial to our well-being. Perhaps the most important relationship of all is the one we have with ourselves.

Intimacy

> *Among men, sex sometimes results in intimacy;*
> *among women, intimacy sometimes results in sex.*
> —BARBARA CARTLAND

> *The opposite of loneliness is not togetherness,*
> *it's intimacy.*
> —RICHARD BACH

True intimacy (into-me-see) comes from allowing ourselves to be vulnerable, opening up and sharing what we are going through, and letting others in. We often hide our feelings because we are ashamed of them, feel needy if we express them, or think that we are the only ones who feel this way. It is only by opening up to someone else authentically that we can really connect.

Yes, anyone can read our Facebook status and know what we are up to, but we rarely post what we are really *feeling*. Social media is great for sharing information and keeping in touch, but it is not a tool that promotes intimacy, necessarily. I can post a blog on my Facebook page, and give readers a deeper insight into my thoughts and feelings, but true intimacy doesn't come through a computer screen or a text message. The feelings are much too complicated and personal to be effectively expressed through those mediums, and communication requires give and take—more than a comment or a "like" can produce.

Intimacy encourages us to take a risk, and allow ourselves to authentically share what we are feeling. Have you ever had this thought? "I want to call my friend, but I haven't talked to her in a while, and I am calling now because I am struggling. I can't call just to dump my problems on her again.

I should wait until I'm feeling happier." Here's a tip for you—that is precisely when you should reach out to someone in your life. Friends are not just there for the good times, and they want to be allowed in when we are going through something difficult. That is what true intimacy is. There is also a big difference between sharing openly and "dumping" a pile of complaints on someone.

A friend disclosed to me once that she had been avoiding being in touch because, "I am your funny friend. The one who makes you laugh, and lightens the mood, and I just haven't been feeling that way lately." I was surprised at how strong my reaction was to this. I was actually angry that she had shut me out when she was going through something difficult and needed me the most. Once she was open about what was going on, it made it easier for me to share my struggles, and we had one of the deepest and most meaningful conversations we have ever had. That wouldn't have happened if she hadn't been able to share her fears and insecurities.

So often in life we put on a happy face, push down our real feelings, and wear a mask that hides from the outside world (and even those closest to us) what is really going on. Every time we do this, we miss an opportunity to truly connect with another human being. Perhaps the most surprising thing about vulnerability is that it rarely goes unreciprocated. When we open up about something in our lives that is causing us pain, it gives others permission to do the same.

Think about all the times you have felt a certain way, but felt scared to express it for whatever reason. So instead, you make an assumption about what is really going on, you beat yourself up for your role, or more likely, you make someone else wrong for "making you" feel this way.

Sometimes we don't share because we think that what we have to say will hurt someone's feelings, or make them angry or push them away. But when we share authentically, without blame or judgment, we open up an opportunity for a deeper connection. How much better would our relationships be if rather than suppressing our feelings or morphing them into something else—most anger comes from a place of hurt—we just shared them in the moment, with as much clarity and vulnerability as we could?

As an alternative to exploding in anger and blaming someone else for not calling when the person said he or she would, imagine yourself saying, "I was really hurt that you didn't call yesterday. Even though our plans were vague, we had agreed to spend the day together, and I am sad that we missed out on that time with each other." Does it feel like weakness to "let someone off the hook" in this way? Think for a minute about what your response to a statement like the one above might be. Then consider what your comeback would look like if you had heard this instead. "You are such a jerk! We had plans yesterday, and you totally blew me off! Did you think I had nothing better to do than sit around and wait for you? I can't even believe I am friends with you. You are so insensitive."

Both statements come from the same feelings, but the first is more authentic and feels *way* scarier because it comes from a place of vulnerability. The second masquerades as coming from a place of strength, which feels safer to us. One puts the other person on the defensive, creating distance, while the other allows an opening for not just a more civil discussion, but a more generous one.

Try This

Who Are You Pretending to Be?

Take out your journal or a piece of paper and write about who you are pretending to be. What masks do you wear? What characteristics do you take on? And what strengths do you pretend? Next, write about who you really are, what you love the most, and those characteristics that may feel like weakness or vulnerabilities. Don't worry about getting this right. There is no such thing. Just allow your pen to flow, and you may be surprised what comes out. Two of the most important questions we face in our life are: Who are you? What do you want? This exercise will give you a start in answering the first better.

Human nature is to "protect ourselves," through saving face, wearing a mask, and playing strong. It takes far more courage and strength to allow ourselves to be vulnerable by expressing what we are really feeling. Practice it the next time you find yourself in a situation like this. Once you see what happens when you respond differently, you will be hooked because of the results you create. It is only through allowing ourselves to feel vulnerable that we can create the kind of deep connection we crave.

Can you remember the last time you allowed yourself to be vulnerable?

What did it feel like? Who was it with?

What would it take for you to create more authentic moments like this in your life?

Soul Mates

A soul mate is someone who has locks that fit our keys, and keys to fit our locks. When we feel safe enough to open the locks, our truest selves step out and we can be completely and honestly who we are; we can be loved for who we are and not for who we're pretending to be. Each unveils the best part of the other. No matter what else goes wrong around us, with that one person we're safe in our own paradise.
—Richard Bach

A loving relationship is one in which the loved one is free to be himself—to laugh with me, but never at me; to cry with me, but never because of me; to love life, to love himself, to love being loved. Such a relationship is based upon freedom and can never grow in a jealous heart.
—Leo Buscaglia

"You complete me." Didn't we all melt when this phrase was uttered in *Jerry McGuire?* The idea of finding our one and only soul mate is so appealing. We want that! Someone who gets where we're coming from and can finish our sentences sounds like just what the doctor ordered. I am a huge fan of the rom com, and another movie from the 1990s that had me searching for my soul mate was *Only You*, starring Marisa Tomei and Robert Downey Jr. Tomei's character finds herself romping around the world chasing the man a childhood Ouiji board session predicted she would marry. I loved the legend in this film about how our souls are broken in two at birth and we are destined to spend our lives searching for our other half.

How sad is it that most of us don't feel whole and complete already? Are we really waiting for someone else to complete us? If two people are already whole and complete and then come together, the two of you can create something magical that wouldn't be possible without the other. That's what I'm talking about!

You have heard it before, and it's true. You can't count on someone else to make you happy. Too often, we seek love from another because we feel broken or damaged or incomplete in some way and we think getting someone else to love us will heal all of that. "You complete me." The opposite is actually true. Heal yourself, love yourself, find happiness, and then you will attract the right person into your life.

Don't get hung up on the idea that there is one perfect person for you either. This keeps us lonely and separate. There could be many people who fulfill you at different stages of your life. We have all had many relationships that were significant and important in helping us learn something we needed to know. We didn't marry all of them, and even if we did, it might not have lasted forever. Be aware of dismissing someone for artificial reasons or expecting perfection, which doesn't exist. It doesn't serve to think of any relationship as a mistake. Each one taught us something that propelled us further along our path.

I have two close friends who both told me they married men who were so far from their "ideal." Why? Because they fell in love with them and realized their idealized version of a man didn't exist, or wasn't worth holding out for when the real thing—which came in bodies with extra pounds, less than hoped for levels of ambition, or with a touch of geekiness—was so much better.

This doesn't mean you won't find one person and get married and spend your entire life with him or her, but just allow yourself to be open, receive what each person is offering, surrender the need to control things, and let go of attachment to a particular outcome. Can you just be present and really feel whatever you're feeling in the moment without worrying about where it's going? That is so difficult for me, as I recently recognized that I don't typically even go on a date with someone unless I think I can marry him. This presents a few problems. First, my friends wouldn't be happily married right now unless they'd gone on a first date with their guys. Two, the expectation that places on the guys I do go out with must be palpable, and probably not that attractive.

A decade or so after those rom com films, I have a much different view on love, and soul mates as well. I definitely believe in the idea of experiencing a soul connection with someone. This is predicated on the idea of reincarnation, and the fact that our souls have met before in previous lives. This means we don't have just one soul mate, but potentially many. You know that feeling of instant connection you have with some people that you just can't explain? That's it.

Elizabeth Gilbert said in *Eat, Pray, Love*, "People think a soul mate is your perfect fit, and that's what everyone wants. But a true soul mate is a mirror, the person who shows you everything that is holding you back, the person who brings you to your own attention so you can change your life."

I believe that relationships (all of them) are meant to teach us something about ourselves, expose us to new ideas, and help us see our own limiting beliefs, so Gilbert's idea resonates. This is why love is not always joyous all the time, and do we honestly expect it to be? By the way, it shouldn't be misery either. Love exists somewhere in-between, where we feel safe enough to share what makes us feel vulnerable, and honest about what causes us pain in the relationship.

I met a Scottish man at a spiritual seminar, and within a few days I was convinced he was "the one." I had a powerful vision (not something that happens to me a lot) of me marrying a man in a kilt, and felt an instant connection with him I couldn't explain.

We met on 11-11-11, a date I had marked in my calendar months before with the words, "Do Something Cool Today." The seminar leader lauded the date as auspicious too, saying it signified the opening of doors for us to walk through into a new life we are creating for ourselves. I like this quote from Bruce Fenton about the significance of the number 11: "I am another yourself, and you are another myself. Each is one. All are one. There is only one." I recently heard Arielle Ford, author of *The Soulmate Secret*, describe two soul mates coming together as not 1+1=2, but 1+1=11 because of the impact that kind of love can have not just on the happy couple, but on the world.

All of this symbolism drew me in, and the initial attraction we felt has been enough to keep us connected over the distance of time and space. Three years later, we are still Skyping every two weeks, and we have seen each other a few times as well. Our relationship is not romantic, but this man from Scotland is definitely a soul mate. We have served as mirrors for each other, and have been able to share incredible things that have helped us both to heal in many ways. Elizabeth Gilbert suggests that this is not the person you end up with, but the person who prepares you for the one. I don't know what will happen between us in the future, but I do know I am worthy of someone who can give me his whole heart, and so is he. I have put a lot of faith in all the symbolism around our meeting date, and the vision I had, but I'm no longer attached to a particular outcome. I am so grateful to have him in my life, and for the healing that is a hallmark of this relationship.

> In a completely interesting sidebar, Emily Hine's spiritual surgery occurred on 11-11-11 in San Diego, the same city where my seminar took place. We didn't yet know each other, and we both lived in other places, but found ourselves in the same city experiencing momentous events on the same day!

What does the term "soul mate" signify for you?

Are you looking for your other half, or do you recognize your wholeness now?

What have you learned from various relationships through the years? Can you see them differently through that context?

Stop Feeling Guilty and Forgive Yourself

Guilt can quickly turn into regret and self-pity. The only way out is through acceptance and forgiveness.
—UNKNOWN

*Your greatest treasure hides behind your self-loathing.
Love it out of hiding.*
—PAMELA MILES

*Forgiveness of yourself is impossible until you stop
longing for a better past.*
—UNKNOWN

Another single survivor said to me recently, "I just can't accept the fact that I somehow caused my cancer." She was confronted by my personal beliefs about finding the root emotional causes of illness in order to better understand and eradicate it from my body. This concept is perhaps the most difficult to explain and to conceptualize. I tried that day to explain to my friend that I don't believe I "caused" my cancer either, but I felt at a loss to put into words the complexity of this idea.

When I was first learning about the Law of Attraction and the power of manifesting, I told an intuitive once that I was afraid I had manifested cancer. She is the one who first helped me get a handle on my own fears and guilt around this concept by telling me we are all manifesting things all the time, and mostly, this is not a conscious act. "If you did manifest it, you did so for a reason," she said, "so stop beating yourself up about it. That does no good."

It is difficult to conceive that there may be some underlying emotional state that causes events in our lives from breakups to accidents and even illness. Most of us would rather not take responsibility for those events, preferring instead to see them as random. Feeling responsible can also make us feel guilty.

Guilt is a powerful emotion, and there are two distinct sides to it. Feeling guilty about something we have done consciously, or even unconsciously, to hurt others will serve us in choosing to do things differently in the future. All too often, though, we feel guilty for no useful reason, and for things that are beyond our control, such as hunger, homelessness, or global warming. Although our actions can impact these, we certainly are not completely responsible for them. This feeling of guilt may spur us to action, or it might just cause us undue stress.

The same is true for our personal issues. Believing that something unconscious inside of us created them can cause us guilt rather than simply acting as a catalyst to help us change an unhealthy pattern. The former isn't useful, but the latter is. When we can change the beliefs that created the pattern, the problem is no longer needed. It was really just there to get our attention anyway. Louise Hay says, "Chronic patterns of self-hate, guilt, and self-criticism raise the body's stress levels and weaken the immune system."

This quote from *The Healing Power of Illness*, by Dr. Ruediger Dahlke and Thorwald Dethlefsen, explains this concept better than I have been able to: "Once people have grasped the difference between illness and symptom, their basic attitude and approach to illness becomes transformed at a stroke. No longer do they see the symptom as the great enemy, which it is their highest goal to resist and destroy. Instead they discover in the symptom a partner capable of helping them to discover what they lack and so to overcome their current illness. At this point the symptom becomes a kind of teacher, helping us take responsibility for our own development and the growth of our consciousness—a teacher, though, who can show great severity and harshness should we fail to respect what is in fact our highest law. Illness knows only one goal: to make us become whole."

I met a woman recently who was dealing with a variety of health issues. As a young mother, she didn't let them slow her down, and literally kept doing laundry while experiencing a stroke. She knew something was wrong, but told herself she couldn't stop caring for her family. Luckily, when I met her, she was taking time for herself at a healing facility focused on mind–body–spirit. For her sake, and that of her family, I hope she can learn to create healthier patterns in her life back at home as well.

I have been exploring emotional patterns through energy healing, and one of the issues I have struggled with is the idea of being alone. I have rarely had a romantic relationship that lasted for more than a few months, and I have made a great deal out of the fact that I am in my 40s and still single. I shared recently in a healing session that I was afraid I would never find true love. It has often been my biggest fear.

The healer I was working with suggested that I have chosen to be alone for so long to learn to love myself. When we don't value ourselves, he said, we seek recognition, admiration, and love from the outside world in disproportionate levels to make up for our own sense of lack. We can over-give in order to receive in return that which is missing. When we truly love ourselves, we take the time for self-care. We drop the judgment. We listen to our inner guidance system and trust ourselves rather than doing what we feel is expected of us from others. We acknowledge our own gifts, and share them with the world. We know what we are worthy of, and don't accept less.

Try This

Examine What You Can Forgive Yourself For

For what do you experience guilt? What do you blame yourself for? What kinds of things do you say to yourself that you wouldn't allow others to say to you? Explore these questions through a meditation exercise. Sit comfortably and read each question. Allow it to sink into your psyche and just be with it for one to five minutes. What comes up? Take notes if you like. Do each question in turn.

Release and Forgive: Once you have explored these past experiences, sit comfortably again, breathe deeply, and say out loud: "I forgive myself for any thoughts, feelings, and actions that don't serve my highest good, and I release any guilt I have about them."

Do this exercise as often as necessary to bring up and release guilt. Forgiveness is a constant practice. We often focus on the importance of forgiving others, but forgiving ourselves is key as well.

What have you felt guilty about that you can do something about?

Where have you carried guilt for things you weren't responsible for? What can you do to release that guilt?

Loving Yourself

To love yourself right now, just as you are, is to give yourself heaven.
Don't wait until you die. If you wait, you die now.
If you love, you live now.
—ALAN COHEN

You must love yourself before you love another. By accepting yourself and fully being what you are, your simple presence can make others happy. You yourself, as much as anybody in the entire universe, deserve your love & affection.
—BUDDHA

Tamika was diagnosed with cervical cancer at 25. Her mom was with her at the appointment, and when the doctor told her she had cancer, she didn't believe him. Because she didn't know anyone else who had been affected, she thought the doctors must have it wrong. Feeling alone and embarrassed about her diagnosis is what led her to found Tamika & Friends, a nonprofit organization whose mission is to educate people about cervical cancer and its links to human papillomavirus (HPV).

Living in D.C. with her dream job as a television producer, Tamika thought about going home to be with her family during treatment. She decided to stay instead, and says her friends were great and totally there for her, but couldn't take time off to be with her during treatment. This is the case for many single, young adults who get cancer and do end up back with their families.

"I had to grow up fast and learn to make decisions on my own," she said. "Life and death decisions on the emotional roller coaster are tough." One of these decisions was one she agonized over—whether or not to have a hysterectomy. Still unmarried, she knew she wanted kids someday, and didn't know what to do. Freezing eggs or embryos was expensive and not covered by insurance. Eventually, Tamika did have the radical surgery, and knew she was giving up her chance to have a family of her own.

Two years after treatment, Tamika finally felt ready to date again. "Right away, I would say, 'My name is Tamika. I have cancer, and I can't have kids,'" she said. "I disclosed way too much too soon, and my friends were good enough to tell me that I should wait until the person was worthy enough to even know this intimate information about me. This was good advice."

At one point she even gave up on the idea that marriage was possible for her. She stayed with people for far too long who weren't right for her because they were willing to accept her baggage and she felt as if she couldn't reject them. Finally, things began to shift.

"I knew I couldn't have kids and that was OK. I was happy with myself and my life," she says. As soon as she really loved herself and accepted the situation as it was, things began changing for her. "I realized I couldn't blame my weight or my survivor status for why I was single," she said. "That was a story. I had to find the right person for me, but I also had to *be* the right person. I wasn't willing to settle, and it was worth waiting for."

Tamika is newly married to someone that she dated before she was diagnosed and briefly after as well. She says the timing wasn't right the first time around because he wanted to get married and she wanted her freedom. Six years later, a friend encouraged her to contact him. She was worried about reaching out because she had rejected him twice before. When he didn't return her first call, she tried again a few months later.

"We've been joined at the hip ever since," she said. "We are the happiest we've ever been, and for us, it really is like picking up where we left off. We know who we are and what we want, and it just works. I'm not settling. He is who I want 100 percent, and he accepts me as I am. He also has a daughter from a previous marriage, so I get the experience of being a mom as well. This is more than I could have asked for, and I feel so blessed."

Tamika's Advice:

1. Love yourself!

2. Get negative people out of your life.

3. Just because you're single doesn't mean anything about you. You're not a loser!

4. Even when you feel like there's no one out there for you, it's not true.

5. I really believed there was someone out there for me. I used to joke that he was just lost, and I needed to send some bigger smoke signals. You have to believe and be hopeful.

6. On one hand, you shouldn't focus on dating too much, but if you want a mate, it has to be a priority. You can't sit home, and you have to be positive.

Sometimes it isn't clear what loving ourselves looks like. This concept encompasses a number of different aspects of who we are: what we look like, how we feel about ourselves, the value we perceive in our own contributions. Loving ourselves can encompass self-acceptance, self-esteem, and self-forgiveness. It can involve cutting ourselves some slack, listening to our own inner guidance, and practicing self-care.

For nearly a year, I did a journaling exercise each morning that entailed making lists related to both of the topics in the following exercise. I immersed myself in exploring the concept of self-love, and passed out stickers at Burning Man one year that said: "Love yourself and you'll never be alone." With that idea, we've come full-circle. Feeling alone is far worse than having cancer, but I've realized that I am the most important person in my life. It's the same for you: you are the most important person in your life. Having a good relationship with me is the basis for everything else.

Try This

Explore what you love most about yourself, and what you love yourself enough to do for YOU.

I Love About Me:

- My long eyelashes
- My blue eyes
- My giving nature
- My love of reading and writing
- My ability to make friends

NOTE: Try not to have all of these be physical traits, perceived strengths, or personality traits each day, but rather a mix of all three.

I Love Myself Enough to:

- Eat healthy food
- Exercise regularly
- Take a walk each morning
- Schedule time in my calendar for myself
- Spend time with friends two to three times a week

NOTE: These should also be a mix of physical, emotional, mental, and social/relational promises. These don't have to be things you already do religiously (though some should), but more aspirational in nature.

While this exercise is a great starting place for exploring what you love about you, eventually it is important to get that you are worthy of love not because of the things on the list, but for no reason at all—just because you are here. As I deepened my spiritual practice it was helpful to me to experience myself as the divine experiences me, and to really deeply feel the sentiment that appeared on a t-shirt I once saw: "I know I'm somebody because God don't make no junk." When I am having a tough time finding something to love about me, I imagine how my creator sees me, and get present to the reason I was put on the planet, and what I have to offer through spirit.

As I have explored the concept of self-love, one of the ways I have decided to express love for myself is in not doing anything I don't want to do. At first glance, this seems impossible. Certainly we all do things we don't love every day. How this has played out for me is in setting boundaries, sometimes changing my perspective about something rather than bailing on the activity itself, and letting go of much of my sense of obligation about things.

How this looks in reality is that I bless my bills now rather than being worried about them, being thankful that the money is there to pay them, or knowing that it will show up somehow. In other words, trusting that I'm being taken care of, and that even if I have to pay only a part of that hospital bill now, the rest will be there next month or the month after.

I sometimes change my mind about doing something that I had committed to, which gives me a few options. Request something different (can we go to a movie instead of ice skating), request to postpone to another time (Can we go next weekend instead? Some things have come up today that are making it difficult to keep my commitment.), or change my attitude (I know it doesn't sound fun, but once I get there, I will enjoy it). I recognize much better now when I am doing something out of a feeling of obligation to someone else or a sense that I "should" do it and not because I really want to, and I really check in with myself before committing in the first place.

I focus on doing work that really fulfills me instead of work that pays the bills, knowing that I will be more engaged and contribute better when I do, and that the fear of taking a job only for the money brings negative energy that doesn't serve me or my mission. I rest when I feel the need to rest, knowing that I will be able to work better if I am well rested and feeling my best.

There is another huge aspect of loving yourself that involves loving and accepting your body. For all of its perceived flaws, scars, tumors, cell mutations, or difficulties, our bodies do amazing things every day that we rarely take the time to recognize, much less appreciate. Breathing, digesting, moving, and eliminating what we don't need. Our bodies are incredible pieces of complex machinery that serve us powerfully, and you would never know it by the way we often talk about them.

"I hate my flabby thighs." "I wish this zit would go away already." "That mole on my shoulder or hair on my chin is disgusting." We say terrible things about our body, and then we expect it to keep on working well for us. Bruce Lipton's book, *The Biology of Belief*, illustrates how much our individual cells absorb the thoughts that we think and the things that we say.

Try This

What Would It Look Like to Love Your Body?

There are a couple of exercises to help you begin to do this. Start where you can and work your way up to loving your body in some way on a daily basis.

Look into a mirror—right into your own eyes and say some of the things you wrote down in the earlier exercise that you love about your body. On an even higher level, make it a habit to say "I love you" to yourself every time you look into a mirror.

When you are in the shower soaping yourself up or putting on lotion, caress all the different parts of your body and say "I love you" as you do so. A woman shared recently that after several months of doing this and truly feeling love for herself and her body as she did so, an ugly, ropy scar on her leg disappeared. You may not have such dramatic external results, but your cells will thank you for sending them loving thoughts for a change.

How much do you love yourself? What does that concept mean to you?

How can you begin to love yourself more?

What can you do to demonstrate your love for you?

There was a moment in time for me in which I just got how much I am loved; not only by my friends and family, but by me, and by God, who I believe is a part of me as well. I recognized how much love is available to me, and to all of us, if we can just allow it in. Love is everywhere, and recognizing it and embracing it only allows more of it to wash over you, especially in those times when you need it the most.

Feeling alone *is* far worse than having cancer, but you don't ever have to feel that way. Love yourself, and you'll never be alone.

You Are Divine

*Nor shall derision prove powerful against those
who listen to humanity or those who follow in the footsteps
of divinity, for they shall live forever. Forever.*
—KHALIL GIBRAN

*If you have anything really valuable to contribute to the world it will
come through the expression of your own personality, that single spark
of divinity that sets you off and makes you different from every other
living creature.*
—BRUCE BARTON

All the themes in this book so far culminate in this single idea of recognizing your own divinity. You are a piece of God, creator, Universe. It has taken
a great deal of time for me to see my own divinity, and to accept the truth
of who I am. And cancer provided rocket fuel for my spiritual process. I
probably would have gotten here eventually, but facing my own mortality
helped me see the truth of my immortality. It led me to seek healing, and

wholeness as my natural state of being. And for that I will always be so grateful for the experience of having had cancer three times. Really, really grateful.

Wholeness

You are all things. Denying, rejecting, judging or
hiding from any aspect of your total being creates pain and
results in a lack of wholeness.
—Joy Page

Pay mind to your own life, your own health, and wholeness.
A bleeding heart is of no help if it bleeds
to death.
—Frederick Buechner

I have had a difficult time always acknowledging my wholeness, the perfect state of being that is me as an expression in the world. I have defaulted instead at times of stress and discomfort to the idea that something is wrong. The situation is wrong, my feelings are wrong, someone else is wrong or most damaging of all, something is wrong with me.

Paul's letter to the Corinthian's, one of the most famous verses of the Bible in Chapter 13, is read at many weddings for what it says about love. This portion applies to my idea of recognizing our wholeness: *When I was a child, I spoke as a child, I understood as a child, I thought as a child; but when I became a man, I put away childish things. For now we see in a mirror, dimly, but then face to face. Now I know in part, but then I shall know just as I also am known.*

As we learn about ourselves and find our places in the world, we are like innocent children, we don't see the fullness of who we really are. From that place of growth, we will make mistakes, and we will hopefully learn from those mistakes and choose something different the next time we are faced with a similar feeling or circumstance. If, instead, we make ourselves wrong or feel guilty, we increase our own suffering. If we make others wrong or bad, we increase our sense of separation from the other whole, complete, and perfect beings who inhabit this planet with us. When we see through a mirror dimly, we just haven't attained the full knowledge of who we are, but as we do, we see face to face, and then as we know the truth of who we are, we allow others to experience the divinity we have to offer the wider world.

One of my favorite quotes from Marianne Williamson also sums up this idea beautifully:

> *Our deepest fear is not that we are inadequate.*
> *Our deepest fear is that we are powerful beyond measure.*
> *It is our light not our darkness that most frightens us.*
> *We ask ourselves, who am I to be brilliant, gorgeous,*
> *talented and fabulous?*
>
> *Actually, who are you not to be?*
> *You are a child of God.*
> *Your playing small does not serve the world.*
> *There's nothing enlightened about shrinking so that other*
> *people won't feel insecure around you.*
>
> *We were born to make manifest the glory of*
> *God that is within us.*
>
> *It's not just in some of us; it's in everyone.*
> *And as we let our own light shine, we unconsciously give*
> *other people permission to do the same.*
>
> *As we are liberated from our own fear,*
> *Our presence automatically liberates others.*

When we step into the wholeness of who we really are, we recognize our own divinity and that of everyone around us. Our freedom to be ourselves, to set boundaries, to practice self-care, to fully express our feelings and to allow others to do the same, provides an opening for everyone to rise to a new level of consciousness. It creates life at an entirely new level.

I recently began dating someone with a similar level of spiritual understanding as me. Because I hadn't necessarily sought out spiritual people to date in the past, this felt exciting. We practiced yoga together and felt comfortable with each other from the very beginning. I knew I didn't have to try to impress him or pretend to be anything that I wasn't. As we spent more time together it became clear that while I was very spiritually in sync with this man, I wasn't romantically attracted to him. I began to worry a bit about what I needed to do about this situation. Should I say something? Would my feelings change? Grow? There was no pressure from him to do anything I was uncomfortable with, so I decided to keep spending time with him, because I really did enjoy his company.

After a date one night, I sensed something different in the way he was approaching me, and I asked him what was wrong. He said, "I had hoped this relationship would have that spark of romance that I've been looking for, and I'm sad that it doesn't." I told him I was sad about that too. There was only a tiny amount of discomfort in having this conversation, and absolutely no blame or awkwardness of any kind. It was so mature, affirming, and supportive. We agreed that we liked each other a lot and would like to remain friends, but that romance probably wasn't in our future. This is what wholeness calls forth.

Wholeness is the goal for physical health as well; however, wholeness does not imply that we are fully intact physically—without missing parts or physical scars. Rather, wholeness refers to that state of mind, body, and spirit being in sync, for each influences the other. When there is a defect in our thinking or in our emotions, it will eventually influence our physical bodies. This can be as simple as a common cold, back pain, or a rash, or as serious as a heart attack, chronic illness, or cancer. The illness is simply the symptom pointing us to explore and heal the disconnect.

Lissa Rankin, MD, expresses this as the whole health cairn that encompasses the major categories of love, service, pleasure, and gratitude as being essential components of a healthy life. Within those categories, she includes physical health, mental health, money, environment, creativity, sexuality, spirituality, work/life purpose, relationships, and something she calls the inner pilot light, the intuitive part of our higher selves. This is how she describes it in her blog: "Your Inner Pilot Light is that ever-radiant, always-sparkly, 100 percent authentic, totally effervescent spark that lies at the core of you. Call it your essential self, your divine spark, your Christ consciousness, your Buddha nature, your higher self, your soul, your wise self, your intuition, or your inner healer."

Healing

Healing comes when we choose to walk away from the darkness
and move toward a brighter light.
—DIETER F. UCHTDORF

When our eyes see our hands doing the work of our hearts, the circle of
Creation is completed inside us, the doors of our souls fly open and love
steps forth to heal everything in sight.
—MICHAEL BRIDGE

What does it mean to be healthy? How do we define healing? What is the difference between the two? The World Health Organization took the traditional definition of health—the absence of physical or psychological pain—one step further and said it is complete physical, mental, and social well-being. Healing, meanwhile, literally means to make whole. Are you sensing a theme here?

Much of modern medicine is focused on defining and alleviating symptoms in both the physical and emotional senses. We take drugs to make us *feel* better, but not to heal us. In a world that makes so many demands on our time, and requires our full focus, alleviating symptoms so we can still function is totally necessary, but if we want to heal what ails us, pharmaceuticals can't do it. It is easy to ask our health care providers to give us something that will help us continue to maintain our incredibly unbalanced and unhealthy lifestyles. High cholesterol medication so we can keep eating cheeseburgers, decongestants and cough medicine so we can work through our colds, and antidepressants to help us appear and feel more "normal" as we go about life.

I am not knocking people who take this route. It is the simplest, most straightforward, and least time-consuming way to deal with illness, and I have used it myself many, many times. Most of us have never been taught that there is another way. The body, mind, and spirit all have incredibly powerful self-healing mechanisms, but they require us to be in a relaxed state, and for many of us, that can seem like a luxury we just don't have time for.

I work from home, have a completely flexible schedule most of the time, don't have kids or a husband to distract me, have full mobility, and rarely face any detrimental effects from cancer, and I still struggle with balancing my emotions, finding time to be physically active and putting my needs first. Bernie Siegel, MD, said in his book *Love, Medicine and Miracles* that those of us who put everyone else's needs ahead of our own are usually the ones who end up with cancer. I took that to heart, and I do a much better job of taking care of myself now than I used to. Having a significant motivation certainly helps this process.

The fight or flight response, which was developed to help us flee from wild animals in hunter-gatherer times, is now triggered on average 50 times a day by such common thoughts, beliefs, and feelings as loneliness, pessimism, work stress, fear of the future, financial concerns, and relationship worries, according to Rankin. We don't have to actually BE in any danger. Just thinking that we may be someday can set off alarm bells in our nervous systems. It reminds me of the long list of personal defects Sally shares with

Harry in the movie that bore their names: "I'm difficult. I'm too structured. I'm completely closed off. And I'm gonna be forty." To the last statement, Harry asks, "When?" And Sally responds, "Someday." That someday, out in our future that we are worried about can cause us health problems today.

If we want to be whole healthy human beings, we can look at illness (symptoms) as a signal that something is wrong, and we can choose to heal that something rather than masking it with alcohol, drugs (prescription or not), or other forms of unhealthy escape. This takes a little more time, energy, and focus. Louise Hay offers a great directory of common illnesses and their emotional roots in her book *You Can Heal Your Life*, but often healing is as simple as taking better care of ourselves, putting ourselves first, and focusing on what we need to be balanced and healthy. It's balancing the doing part of ourselves with the being part, and recognizing that, after all, we are human beings and not human doings.

Sometimes the "cure" is forced upon us when we have no choice but to rest with an injury or an illness. This is why I will always see my cancer not as a burden, but as a complete blessing. Cancer forced my hand. It made me slow down, take stock of what wasn't working, reach out to my community for support, recognize how loved I am, quit my job, change my diet, and find a better way. What if we took more time for things we love regularly? Would we be less likely to get sick in the first place? Whether it's a sick day, a vacation, more time with friends and family, yoga, time in nature, a good book or a massage, we need to know what triggers our own relaxation response and make those activities a priority. Relaxation is a precursor to allowing the parasympathetic nervous system to heal us.

It is gratifying to hear stories of people battling serious illness who heal the major relationships and negative patterns in their lives even if, ultimately, they don't survive. It is possible to find healing, even without total health. There are also many stories of people who when diagnosed with a terminal illness quit their miserable jobs or left their unfulfilling marriages, started living the lives they wanted to live and suddenly got well. You can read more about them online at the Spontaneous Remission Project or in Kelly Turner's book *Radical Remission*. When we can heal the guilt, shame, and unworthiness that may lie hidden under an outwardly happy countenance, the miraculous can happen—and not just in terms of whatever disease we are dealing with—truly, our lives can take on new purpose and meaning.

Some people struggle with this concept, because if we truly can heal ourselves, and I haven't been able to do it, does it mean that I am to blame for still being sick? Absolutely not! We are all doing the best that we can with the information we have available to us at the moment. As we learn more, we can do more. Transformation is a process. Beating ourselves up for wherever we happen to be now is counterproductive.

There is a delicate balance in all of life between being satisfied with and grateful for what is, and also seeking for what could be. Buddhism calls it the middle way, and the Buddha described it as a life lived between the extremes of self-denial and self-indulgence. The Tao describes it in the balance between yin and yang and describes the two forces depicted in the black and white image as complementary rather than opposing. All of these philosophies point to the idea that light can't exist without darkness, and yet we often curse one and seek the other. The balance point is where the magic is.

Oneness

The whole of planet Earth is a sacred site. All the people are the chosen
people, and the purpose of our lives is a spiritual one. May we care for
each other, and for the earth, for everything relates to everything else.
Feeling this oneness, may we radiate the light of love and kindness that all
may live in unity and peace.
—Radha Sahar

Once you are able to look at another human being and see no difference
at all, there is no need for harmony. For here, there is only oneness.
This is the place the story began. And this is the end toward which all
consciousness now strives to return.
—Buddha

A human being is a part of the whole, called by us, universe, a part
limited in time and space. He experiences himself, his thoughts
and feelings as something separated from the rest, a kind of optical
delusion of his consciousness. This delusion is a kind of prison for us,
restricting us to our personal desires and to affection for a few persons
nearest to us. Our task must be to free ourselves from this prison by
widening our circle of compassion to enhance all living creatures and
the whole of nature in its beauty.
—Albert Einstein

There is a universal consciousness that connects all life from bugs and plants to human beings and star systems. Often called the God connection, this unity is what calls forth our highest good, and inspires us to offer it freely to one another. It is the Namaste energy that says the light (or divine) in me acknowledges and bows to the light in you. This consciousness is embodied in each and every human being, and connects us all to one another. This consciousness is what would have us protect and preserve the plants and animals that share our planet and keep the water, air, and earth as unpolluted as possible.

As a part of my own balancing process, I have spent a great deal of time, energy, and money on my own personal development and growth through attending retreats, reading books, participating in seminars and workshops, and taking various experiential classes. There were times when I felt guilty about all the resources and time I put toward this path, feeling that I should be doing more, giving more, or creating more to benefit others instead. My inquiry led me to become fascinated with quantum physics, and I read a number of books that helped me recognize there was a connection between science and the universal consciousness, and in fact, these were the same thing.

As I built a daily meditation practice, a regular yoga practice, allowed myself to rest, spend time with loved ones, be outside in nature and continue my personal growth, I began to see the impact my development could have on the larger world as I shared what I was learning and experiencing with others. Suddenly it no longer seemed selfish. I even read about numerous studies that have been done on the connections between peace and transcendental meditation. These studies involved a small number of people meditating or praying at the same time, in the same place (notably, Washington, DC, and Israel) and resulting in significant decreases in crime, traffic accidents, deaths, fires, and other indicators of social stress. This helped me recognize that indeed, raising my own consciousness could have profound impacts beyond myself.

I know that we have the power to heal ourselves, and I have been reluctant to share this belief too widely for fear that others would misinterpret and blame themselves for the fact that they were sick, or dismiss what I was saying as a bunch of woo woo fairytale. And at the same time, I know that those who are ready to hear this message and take the time to explore it for themselves will benefit tremendously. I have tried to release any sense of ego to share authentically and vulnerably with you in this book about my own journey in order that it may light the way for others.

I AM

*While I know myself as a creation of God, I am also
obligated to realize and remember that everyone else and
everything else are also God's creation.*
—MAYA ANGELOU

The I AM is a useful pointer; it shows where to seek, but not what to seek. Just have a good look at it. Once you are convinced that you cannot say truthfully about yourself anything except I AM, and that nothing that can be pointed at can be yourself, the need for the I AM is over. You are no longer intent on verbalizing what you are. All definitions apply to your body only and to its expressions. Once this obsession with the body goes, you will revert to your natural state.
—Sri Nisargadatta Maharaj

You can read my Enough Manifesto at the end of the book. In it I share how our own definitions of ourselves are limiting in nature—sister, writer, daughter, vegan, woman. They put us into a box by which any way we can describe ourselves is inadequate. Do these labels even begin to hint at who we really are – spiritual beings having a human experience?

I AM is the full expression of our soul purpose—the reason we came here in a body to begin with. It is about our own unique individualization of the God Consciousness—that thing that we are here to do, and if we don't do it, it won't be expressed in the world. Those limiting beliefs that we carry around keep us from fulfilling that mission. Our fear that we aren't good enough, don't know enough, can't express it correctly, aren't doing it right, might be laughed at, ridiculed, or snubbed keeps us from being our unique manifestation in the world.

I have had to get over myself in order to be a speaker, start a nonprofit, give media interviews as an "expert" in anything, write a blog and a book and speak my truth. There is always the balance between not good enough and arrogance or pride. Walking the middle way has allowed me to share what I believe and be OK with the fact that many will disagree, some will feel threatened and possibly attack me, and others will be inspired to find a better way themselves, and to know that all of those reactions are valid. The trick is to let none of them impact me, either in puffing me up, or in bringing me down.

Seeking this harmony between the Alpha and the Omega aspects of my being has brought me peace, and healing and a recognition of what is left when all of those fears are collapsed: ONLY LOVE.

A Final Note: Love Your Life

Congratulations for reading all the way through to the end. Now that you have realized you are not alone, you have options, you are responsible, you are a survivor, worthy, lovable, inspirational, powerful, loved, and divine. . . what are you going to do with that? You can go back to living the way you were before you discovered all of this about yourself, put this book on the shelf, and forget about it. OR, you can take action to improve your life, your health, and increase your level of happiness.

I challenge you to take some action. Right now. Today. If you haven't done the exercises in the book, go back and do them now. Get a highlighter and go back through the book for the parts you want to remember and apply to your life. Take out a journal and write about what this brought up for you, and how the ideas have changed your thinking. Read the book again and share it with others. Perhaps start a discussion group or a book club to talk about what you learned.

In the blank lines below, I want you to write down ten actions that you will commit to in the next 90 days. It could be to hire a coach, commit to a meditation practice, start a gratitude or loving yourself journal, change your diet, reach out to your community, or any number of other things that will support your health and well-being—your mind, body, and spirit. What are you going to DO?

1. _____

_____

2. _____

_____

3. _____

_____

4. _____

_____

5. _____

_____

6. _____

_____

7. _____

_____

8. _____

_____

9. _____

_____

10. _____

_____

I hope the stories you read of other single survivors like yourself, and their fears, triumphs, and disappointments, helped you feel less alone. That you have recognized how many options you have for treating your cancer and living your life more fully. That you have embraced the idea of taking responsibility for your life, and even learned to embrace your survivor status. That the exercises have helped you take control of creating the kind of inspirational, powerful, and loving life that you deserve. I deeply desire for you to recognize your own value, worth, and uniqueness, and discover how you can share your special gifts with the world. Most of all, I hope you now see that you are truly and completely loved and lovable.

I encourage you to contact me about what you learned, what you wish had been included, what was immediately useful, and what didn't resonate as deeply, what you are struggling with and how I can help. I wrote this book for YOU. It was the book I wished I had when I was diagnosed, and I truly want it to help others. Your feedback will help me improve future editions, and if you want to go deeper in exploring these concepts, I am happy to help with that as well. You can contact me via e-mail at tracy@solosurvivors.com.

I truly wish you an amazing life! I want you to have life, love, health, and happiness, and I am excited to help you achieve the life of your dreams. I would be thrilled to offer you a complimentary, no obligation 30 to 60 minute coaching session by phone or Skype to explore whatever challenges you are facing and to discover how I might be able to support you.

❧ THE ENOUGH MANIFESTO, PART I ❧

~ BY TRACY MAXWELL ~

I AM NOT A COLLECTION OF COMPLAINTS, **SHORTCOMINGS,** MISTAKES, WOUNDS, OR VICES. NOR AM I **A COMPILATION OF SUCCESSES, HONORS,** HAPPY MOMENTS, BREAKTHROUGHS, TRIUMPHS OR JOYS.

I AM NOT MY PAST. NOT MY STORIES.

I AM NOT MY BODY

MY APPEARANCE, MY PHYSICAL SCARS, MY EYE OR HAIR OR SKIN COLOR.

I AM NOT MY **EXPERIENCES,** OR INSIGHTS **OR ILLNESSES.**

I AM NOT MY **FAMILY, OR** SOCIOECONOMIC STATUS **OR OCCUPATION.**

I AM NOT THE HOUSE I LIVE IN OR THE CAR I DRIVE, **THE CLOTHES I WEAR OR THE THINGS I OWN.**

I AM NOT MY HUMILIATIONS, MY TITLES, OR MY AFFILIATIONS. **I AM NOT MY ABILITIES, MY TALENTS OR MY CONNECTIONS.**

I AM NOT MY GENDER, MY RACE, MY SEXUAL ORIENTATION, MY ETHNICITY ❧ **OR EVEN MY DNA.** ❧

I AM NOT MY FINGERPRINT, MY PHOTO, MY FACEBOOK PROFILE, **MY ADDRESS OR** MY LAST NAME.

I AM NOT MY CITY, MY COUNTRY, **MY BODY TYPE,** MY WEIGHT OR **MY AGE.**

I AM NOT MY MARITAL STATUS, **MY HOBBIES,** MY BELIEFS, **MY RELIGION OR** MY FRIENDSHIPS.

I AM NOT THE LABELS YOU GIVE ME, OR THE ONES I GIVE MYSELF. **I AM NOT MY GRIEF OR MY CELEBRATION.** I AM NOT MY CHILDHOOD OR MY ANCESTRY.

I AM NOT WHO YOU THINK I AM. I AM NOT WHO I THINK I AM. **⚜ AND NEITHER ARE YOU. ⚜**

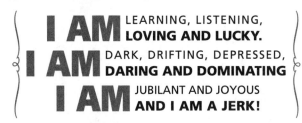

THE ENOUGH MANIFESTO, PART II

BY TRACY MAXWELL

I AM UNIQUE, IMPERFECT, CONSCIOUS, ALIVE, AWAKE AND FREE.
I AM LOVED, DESPISED, INSPIRED, AWED AND ADORED.
I AM SAD, TRUSTING, OPEN, DISAPPOINTED AND SCARED.

I AM LEARNING, LISTENING, **LOVING AND LUCKY.**

I AM DARK, DRIFTING, DEPRESSED, **DARING AND DOMINATING**

I AM JUBILANT AND JOYOUS **AND I AM A JERK!**

I AM ALONE, CONNECTED, OUTGOING, WITHDRAWN,
DESPONDENT, HOPEFUL, GRACIOUS AND DEMANDING.

I AM CONFIDENT **AND** I AM TERRIFIED.

I AM ARROGANT 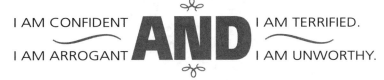 I AM UNWORTHY.

I AM HEALTHY, HAPPY, HOLY, HELPFUL AND HATED.
I AM INTUITIVE, INSTRUCTIVE, INSPIRATIONAL, ILL-PREPARED AND IDIOTIC.

I AM
FORGIVING, TRUSTED,
BEAUTIFUL, UGLY,
PLAIN, COMPLICATED
AND SIMPLE.

I AM
KIND, CONSIDERATE
IGNORANT, OUT-OF-TOUCH
GIVING AND
UNAWARE.

I AM INTERESTED, INQUISITIVE, INTELLIGENT AND ODD.
I AM EVEN-TEMPERED, BELOVED, DISCONNECTED, DISBELIEVING, DEBILITATED AND DETERMINED
I AM SILLY, SERIOUS, SENTIMENTAL AND SUPERFICIAL.

I AM PROUD, AND I AM ASHAMED.
I AM AFRAID, AND I AM PEACEFUL.
I AM DETERMINED, AND I AM ALLOWING.
I AM GRATEFUL, AND I AM LACKING.

I AM ALL, AND I AM NOTHING. AND SO ARE YOU.

I AM.
I AM ENOUGH.

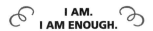

AND SO ARE YOU.

References

Introduction

Klinenberg, Eric. *Going Solo: The Extraordinary Rise and Surprising Appeal of Living Alone.* New York: Penguin, 2012.

Siegel, Bernie S. *Love, Medicine and Miracles.* New York: William Morrow Paperbacks, 1990.

Chapter 1

Klinenberg, *Going Solo.*

Madson, Jenifer. *Living the Promises: Coming to Life on the Road to Recovery.* Newburyport, MA: Red Wheel/Weiser, 2011.

Ornish, Dean. *Love & Survival: Eight Pathways to Intimacy and Health.* New York: Harper-Collins, 1998.

Rankin, Lissa, MD. *Mind Over Medicine: Scientific Proof That You Can Heal Yourself.* Carlsbad, CA: Hay House, 2013.

Spiegel, David. *Living Beyond Limits.* New York: Ballantine Books, 1994.

Chapter 2

Buffart, Laurien M., Jannique G. Z. van Uffelen, Ingrid I. Riphagen, Johannes Brug, Willem van Mechelen, Wendy J. Brown, and Mai JM Chinapaw. "Physical and psychosocial benefits of yoga in cancer patients and survivors, a systematic review and meta-analysis of randomized controlled trials." *BMC cancer* 12, no. 1 (2012): 559.

Campbell, T. Colin. *The China Study: The Most Comprehensive Study of Nutrition Ever Conducted and the Startling Implications for Diet, Weight Loss and Long-Term Health.* Dallas: BenBella Books, 2004.

Crazy, Sexy Cancer documentary, directed by Kris Carr, Cactus Three (Sparta, NJ: Red House Productions, 2007) DVD.

Esselstyn, Rip. *The Engine 2 Diet: The Texas Firefighter's 28-Day Save-Your-Life Plan that Lowers Cholesterol and Burns Away the Pounds.* New York: Grand Central Publishing, 2009.

Fellowes Deborah, Kelly Barnes, and Susie S. M. Wilkinson. "Aromatherapy and Massage for Symptoms Relief in Patients with Cancer." *Cochrane Database of Systematic Reviews,* no. 4 (2008): CD002287. doi: 10.1002/14651858.CD002287 .pub3

Harder, H., L. Parlour, and V. Jenkins. "Randomised controlled trials of yoga interventions for women with breast cancer: a systematic literature review." *Supportive Care in Cancer* 20, no. 12 (2012): 3055–3064.of yoga:

Lipton, Bruce H. *The Biology of Belief: Unleashing the Power of Consciousness, Matter & Miracles.* Carlsbad, CA: Hay House, 2007.

Pachman, Deirdre R., Debra L. Barton, Keith M. Swetz, and Charles L. Loprinzi. "Troublesome symptoms in cancer survivors: fatigue, insomnia, neuropathy, and pain." *Journal of Clinical Oncology* 30, no. 30 (2012): 3687–3696.

Pollan, Michael. *In Defense of Food.* New York: Penguin Press, 2008.

Vickers, Andrew J., Angel M. Cronin, Alexandra C. Maschino, George Lewith, et al. "Acupuncture for Chronic Pain: Individual Patient Data Meta-Analysis." *Archives of Internal Medicine* 172, no. 19 (2012): 1444–1453.

Chapter 3

Emotional Freedom Techniques (EFT), Tapping, www.thetappingsolution.com/blog/tag/nick-ortner

Hay, Louise. *You Can Heal Your Life.* Carlsbad, CA: Hay House Publishing, 1984.

Hine, Emily. Holy Sit (blog), www.holysit.com/p/holy-sit.html

In The Family, documentary, directed by Joanna Rudnick, produced by Joanna Rudnick, Kartemquin Films, and Independent Television Service, 2008.

Pausch, Randy. *The Last Lecture.* New York: Hyperion, 2008.

Rankin, Lissa, MD. *Mind Over Medicine: Scientific Proof That You Can Heal Yourself.* Carlsbad, CA: Hay House, 2013.

Williamson, Marianne. *A Return to Love: Reflections on the Principles of "A Course in Miracles."* New York: Harper One, 1996.

Chapter 4

Collins, Jim. *Good to Great.* New York: Harper Business, 2001.

Swarner, Sean, and Rusty Fisher. *Keep Climbing: How I Beat Cancer and Reached the Top of the World.* New York: Atria Books, 2007.

Chapter 5

Brown, Brene. *Daring Greatly: How the Courage to Be Vulnerable Transforms the Way We Live, Love, Parent and Lead.* New York: Gotham, 2012.

Brene Brown TED Talks:
Vulnerability, http://www.ted.com/talks/brene_brown_on_vulnerability.html
Shame, http://www.ted.com/talks/brene_brown_listening_to_shame.html

DePaulo, Bella. *Singled Out.* New York: St. Martin's Press, 2007.

Moorjani, Anita. *Dying to Be Me: My Journey from Cancer, to Near Death, to True Healing*. Carlsbad, CA: Hay House, 2012.

Chapter 6

Aizer, Ayal A., and Paul L. Nguyen, et al. "Marital Status and Survival in Patients with Cancer." *Journal of Clinical Oncology* 3, no. 31(2013): 3852–3853.

Chapman, Gary D. *The Five Love Languages: The Secret to Love That Lasts*. Chicago: Northfield Publishing, 2009.

Doyle, Laura. *The Surrendered Single*. New York: Touchstone, 2002.

Frobisher, Claire, et al. "Long-Term Population-Based Marriage Rates Among Adult Survivors of Childhood Cancer in Britain." *International Journal of Cancer* 121, no. 4 (2007): 846–855.

Harmon, Katherine "How Important Is Physical Contact with Your Infant?" Scientific American, May 6, 2010. Online version downloaded from: www.scientificamerican.com/article/infant-touch

Luscombe, Belinda. "Who Needs Marriage? A Changing Institution." *Time*, November 18, 2010. Online version downloaded from: http://content.time.com/time/magazine/article/0,9171,2032116,00.html

Rosenthal, Kairol. *Everything Changes*. Hoboken, NJ: Wiley, 2009.

Whitlock, Michelle. *How I Lost My Uterus and Found My Voice*. Bloomington, IN: iUniverse, 2011.

Chapter 7

The Center for Research on the Effects of Television (CRETV). "Television in the Lives of Children." www.ithaca.edu/cretv/research/tv_lives.html

Landmark Worldwide. www.landmarkworldwide.com

Williamson, Marianne. *A Return to Love*.

Chapter 8

Constantine, Andrea, and Lisa Schultz. *How to Bring Your Book to Life This Year: A Guidebook on Writing and Self-Publishing*. Self Publishing Experts, LLC, and CreateSpace, Amazon.com, 2010.

Dooley, Mike. *Leveraging the Universe: Seven Steps to Engaging Life's Magic*. New York: Simon & Schuster, 2011.

Doyle, Laura. *The Surrendered Single*.

Emoto, Masaru. *The Hidden Messages in Water*. New York: Simon & Schuster, 2011.

Frankl, Viktor. *Man's Search for Meaning*. Boston: Beacon Press, 1959.

Gilbert, Elizabeth. *Committed*. New York: Viking Adult, 2010.

Hine, Emily. Holy Sit (blog), http://www.holysit.com/p/holy-sit.html

Is Medicine Killing You? TEDx, Fargo, September 2, 2013, www.youtube.com/
watch?v=EUYLa7MAlPc

Is There Scientific Proof We Can Heal Ourselves? TEDx Talks, December 18, 2012,
www.youtube.com/watch?v=LWQfe__fNbs

Rankin, Lissa, MD. *Mind Over Medicine.*

Chapter 9

Dethlefsen, Thorwald, and Dr. Ruediger Dahlke. *The Healing Power of Illness:
Understanding What Your Symptoms Are Telling You.* London: Vega Books, 2002.

Ford, Arielle. *The Soulmate Secret: Manifest the Love of Your Life with the Law of
Attraction.* New York: Harper One, 2011.

Gilbert, Elizabeth. *Eat, Pray, Love.* New York: Penguin, 2006.

Chapter 10

The Bible. King James Version, 1 Corinthians 13, verse 11.

Braden, Gregg. *The Spontaneous Healing of Belief.* Carlsbad, CA: Hay House, 2008

Rankin, Lissa, MD. *Mind Over Medicine.*

Reiner, Rob and Ephron, Nora. When Harry Met Sally. . .Motion Picture. Directed
by Rob Reiner. New York. Columbia, 1989.

Spontaneous Remission Project, Institute of Noetic Sciences, www.noetic.org/
research/project/online-spontaneous-remission-bibliography-project

Transcendental Meditation Blog, www.tm.org/blog/video/
world-peace-from-the-quantum-level-david-lynch-and-john-hagelin

Turner, Kelly A. *Radical Remission: Surviving Cancer Against All Odds.* New York:
HarperOne, 2014.

Williamson, Marianne. *A Return to Love.*

Zukav, Gary. *The Dancing Wu Li Masters: An Overview of the New Physics.* New
York: HarperOne, 2001.

Resources

Online

Cancer-Related Organizations
General

Athletes for Cancer
Harnessing the healing power of wind and water with the determination of the human spirit. Surf and snow camps.

http://athletes4cancer.org

BAG IT
BAG IT is committed to providing information and education to newly diagnosed individuals with cancer and their families.

http://bagit4u.org

Camp Mak-A-Dream
A cost-free camp for children and young adults with cancer, located in Montana and operated by the Children's Oncology Camp Foundation.

www.campdream.org

Cancer and Careers
Support for people working while trying to manage their cancer and careers.

www.cancerandcareers.org/en

Cancer Care
Professional counseling, facilitated peer support groups, creative workshops, and financial assistance for young adults with cancer.

www.cancercare.org/get_help/special_progs/young_adults.php

Cancer Climber
Offering experiential and motivational adventures and excursions such as extreme mountain climbing and summit tours.

www.cancerclimber.org

Cancer Legal Resource Center
The CLRC provides information and education about cancer-related legal issues.

www.disabilityrightslegalcenter.org/cancer-legal-resource-center

Chemo Angels
The goal of Chemo Angels is to help fuel a positive attitude and aid in the road to recovery.

chemoangels.wix.com/chemo-angels-1

Emerald Heart Foundation
Financial support and other resources for women in effective uninsured alternative cancer treatments.

www.emeraldheart.org

Fertile Action
To help women touched by cancer become mothers.

www.fertileaction.org

Fertile Hope
Provides reproductive health information, support, and hope to cancer patients whose medical treatments present the risk of infertility.

www.fertilehope.org

First Descents
An innovative camp experience for young adults with cancer, offering kayaking, extreme sports, and professional athletics.

www.firstdescents.org

Gilda's Club
Creates welcoming communities of free support for everyone living with cancer—men, women, teens, and children—along with their families and friends.

www.gildasclubdetroit.org (these can be found in many cities)

Imerman Angels
To provide personalized connections that enable one-on-one support among cancer fighters, survivors, and caregivers.

www.imermanangels.org

I'm Too Young for This (Stupid Cancer)
To ensure that no one affected by young adult cancer go unaware of the age-appropriate support resources they are entitled to so they can get busy living.

stupidcancer.org

LifeSpark (Denver)
Provides Reiki and healing touch for cancer patients to help with side effects and support mind, body, and spirit.

http://lifesparknow.org

LIVESTRONG Foundation
Unites and empowers people affected by cancer.

www.livestrong.org

MyLifeLine
To empower patients to build an online support community of family and friends to foster connection, inspiration, and healing.

www.mylifeline.org

Pink Elephant Posse
Finds young women affected by cancer and puts them in the spotlight to be heard, seen, and loved.

http://pinkelephantposse.org

Planet Cancer
Young adult–focused community offering survivor retreat programs, social networking, and online forums with real world advice and inspiring stories.

http://myplanet.planetcancer.org

re org (Denver)
Pairs cancer survivors with massage therapists to work together for a six-month period in order to create lasting change in survivors' bodies and lives following treatment.

www.re-orgdenver.org

Rise Above It
Provides grants and scholarships to young adult survivors and care providers who face financial, emotional, and spiritual challenges.

www.raibenefit.org

SeventyK
Mission is to change cancer care by educating patients, families, and their healthcare providers about age-appropriate treatment and the unique needs of the adolescent and young adult (AYA) cancer patient.

www.seventyk.org

Solo Survivors
Support for singles dealing with cancer. This is not a dating service, but rather a place to feel connected to a larger community of singles who are facing similar challenges for support, sharing, and connection.

www.solosurvivors.com

Tamika & Friends
Dedicated to raising awareness about cervical cancer and its links to HPV, the organization believes that through education, prevention, and treatment, cervical

cancer can be entirely eliminated as communication is far more infectious than HPV.

www.tamikaandfriends.org

Truly Heal
A comprehensive website designed to be the unification of alternative health education for all degenerative diseases.

http://trulyheal.com

Voices of Survivors
Devoted to exploring what "Survivorship" means to the individual "Survivor," whether the individual is recently diagnosed, in-treatment, or post-treatment, in a variety of documentary formats.

http://voicesofsurvivors.org

Young Survivor Coalition
An international network of breast cancer survivors and supporters dedicated to the concerns and issues that are unique to young women and breast cancer.

www.youngsurvival.org

Ovarian Cancer

Colorado Ovarian Cancer Alliance
Provide support and promote awareness and early detection of ovarian cancer through advocacy and education.

www.colo-ovariancancer.org

HERA Women's Cancer Foundation
Stop the loss of women from ovarian cancer.

http://www.herafoundation.org

National Cancer Institute at the National Institutes of Health
Cancer research and training.

www.cancer.gov/cancertopics/types/ovarian

National Ovarian Cancer Coalition
The Coalition is committed to improving the survival rate and quality of life for women with ovarian cancer.

www.ovarian.org

Ovarian Cancer National Alliance
Advancing the interests of women with ovarian cancer.

www.ovariancancer.org

Counselors and Therapists

Ask your hospital or medical practitioners for recommendations first, and then try these sources.

American Association of Sexuality Educators, Counselors and Therapists (AASECT)

www.aasect.org

American Psychology Society (APOS)
apos-society.org

Association of Oncology Social Work (AOSW)

www.aosw.org

Society for Sex Therapy and Research (SSTAR)

www.sstarnet.org

Courses and Programs

A Course in Miracles
www.acim.org

Byron Katie
www.thework.com/index.php

Enneagram
www.enneagraminstitute.com/intro.asp

Emotional Freedom Techniques (EFT), Tapping
http://www.thetappingsolution.com

Feminine Power
http://femininepower.com/online-course/free-online-class

Landmark Worldwide
www.landmarkworldwide.com

The Receiving Project
www.receivingproject.com

Totally Unique Thoughts (Thoughts Become Things)
www.tut.com

Observances

National Cancer Survivors Day

www.ncsd.org

World Cancer Day

www.worldcancerday.org

Books

Inspiration and Motivation

Collins, Jim. *Good to Great*. New York: Harper Business, 2001.

Davis, Nancy. *Lean on Me: Ten Powerful Steps for Moving Beyond Your Diagnosis and Taking Back Your Life*. New York: Fireside, 2006.

Fox, Michael J. *A Funny Thing Happened on the Way to the Future*. New York: Hyperion, 2010.

Cancer, Health, and Wellness

Carr, Kris. *Crazy, Sexy Cancer Tips*. Guilford, CT: Skirt! Publishing, 2007.

Gerson, Max. *A Cancer Therapy*. San Diego, CA: Gerson Institute, 1958.

Hay, Louise. *You Can Heal Your Life*. Carlsbad, CA: Hay House Publishing, 1984.

Moorjani, Anita. *Dying to Be Me: My Journey from Cancer, to Near Death, to True Healing*. Carlsbad, CA: Hay House, 2012.

Pausch, Randy. *The Last Lecture*. New York: Hyperion, 2008.

Quinn, Hollie, and Patrick Quinn. *You Did What? Saying No to Conventional Cancer Treatment*. Peterborough, NH: Cobblestone Publishing, 2010.

Rankin, Lissa, MD. *Mind Over Medicine: Scientific Proof That You Can Heal Yourself*. Carlsbad, CA: Hay House, 2013.

Servan-Schriber, David. *Anti-Cancer*. New York: Viking Press, 2009.

Siegel, Bernie S. *Love, Medicine and Miracles*. New York: William Morrow Paperbacks, 1990.

Spiegel, David. *Living Beyond Limits*. New York: Ballantine Books, 1994.

Swarner, Sean, and Rusty Fisher. *Keep Climbing*. New York: Atria Books, 2007.

Turner, Kelly A., PhD. *Radical Remission: Surviving Cancer Against All Odds*. New York: HarperOne, 2014.

Whitlock, Michelle. *How I Lost My Uterus and Found My Voice*. Bloomington, IN: iUniverse, 2011.

Food

Campbell, T. Colin. *The China Study*. Dallas: BenBella Books, 2004.

Carr, Kris. *Crazy, Sexy Diet*. Guilford, CT: Skirt! Publishing, 2011.

Carr, Kris. *Crazy, Sexy Kitchen: 150 Plant-Empowered Recipes to Ignite a Mouthwatering Revolution*. Carlsbad, CA: Hay House, 2012.

D'Adamo, Peter. *Eat Right for Your Type*. New York: Penguin Books, 1996.

Esselstyn, Rip. *The Engine 2 Diet*. New York: Grand Central Publishing, 2009.

Graham, Tyler, and Drew Ramsey, MD. *The Happiness Diet: A Nutritional Prescription for a Sharp Brain, Balanced Mood and Lean, Energized Body*. New York: Rodale, 2011.

Kingsolver, Barbara. *Animal, Vegetable, Miracle*. New York: Harper, 2007.

Pollan, Michael. *In Defense of Food*. New York: Penguin Press HC, 2008.

Young, Robert O., and Shelley Redford Young. *The pH Miracle: Balance Your Diet, Reclaim Your Health*. New York: Wellness Central, 2003.

Money

Kessel, Brent. *It's Not About the Money*. New York: Harper Collins, 2008.

Northrup, Kate. *Money: A Love Story*. Carlsbad, California: Hay House, 2013.

Roth, Geneen. *Lost and Found*. New York: Viking Penguin, 2011.

Scheinfeld, Robert. *Busting Loose from the Money Game*. Hoboken, NJ: Wiley, 2006.

Williamson, Marianne. *The Law of Divine Compensation: On Work, Money and Miracles*. New York: Harper Collins, 2012.

Personal Growth, Spiritual

Ban Breathnach, Sarah. *Simple Abundance*. New York: Grand Central Publishing, 1996.

Byron, Katie, and Stephen Mitchell. *Loving What Is*. New York: Three Rivers Press, 2003.

Dooley, Mike. *Leveraging the Universe*. New York: Atria Books/Beyond Words, 2011.

Ferris, Timothy. *The Four-Hour Work Week*. New York: Crown Archtype, 2007.

Fox, Michael J. *A Funny Thing Happened on the Way to the Future*. New York: Hyperion, 2010.

Gilbert, Daniel. *Stumbling on Happiness*. New York: Vintage Books, 2007.

Millman, Dan. *Everyday Enlightenment: The Twelve Gateways to Personal Growth*. New York: Grand Central Publishing, 1999.

Palmer, Parker. *A Hidden Wholeness: The Journey Toward an Undivided Life*. San Francisco: Jossey-Bass, 2009.

Palmer, Parker. *Let Your Life Speak: Listening for the Voice of Vocation*. San Francisco: Jossey-Bass, 1999.

Ruiz, Don Miguel. *The Four Agreements*. San Rafael, CA: Amber-Allen Publishing, 1997.

Shalimar, Ilan. *Simple Wisdom: A Thousand Things Went Right Today*. Fort Collins, CO: Your True Nature, Inc, 2003.

Zelenski, Ernie. *The Joy of Not Working*. New York: Ten Speed Press, 1997.

Relationships

Doyle, Laura. *The Surrendered Single*. New York: Touchstone, 2002.

Eckel, Sara. *It's Not You: 27 (WRONG) Reasons You're Single*. New York: Perigee Trade, 2014.

Ford, Arielle. *The Soulmate Secret: Manifest the Love of Your Life with the Law of Attraction*. New York: HarperOne, 2011.

Gilbert, Elizabeth. *Committed*. New York: Viking Adult, 2010.

Ornish, Dean. *Love & Survival: Eight Pathways to Intimacy and Health*. New York: Harper-Collins, 1998.

Woodward-Thomas, Katherine. *Calling in "The One."* New York: Crown Publishing, 2004.

Acknowledgments

There are many people to thank in a situation like this because truly no one ever writes a book or achieves any kind of success alone. There are always those upon whose shoulders we stand, whose advice forwards our thinking, whose encouragement strengthens our resolve, whose support buoys us through the difficult times. It is not possible to properly recognize all who have helped this book come to life through their one-time, occasional, and even constant interaction with me. All those interactions are the very stuff of life that make us all who we are. For each and every one of them, I am grateful.

If you have ever read anything I wrote, heard me on a radio or television interview, interacted with me through social media, taught me in any sort of class or seminar, listened to me cry or celebrated with me, been an audience member in any of my workshops or programs, shared a seat next to me on a plane or on a road trip or in a canoe, learned to swim from me, held my hand through a difficulty, seen something in me that I didn't see in myself, shared your frustration with me, opened your heart to me, held me accountable, made me laugh or laughed with me, given me a hug or supported me, I acknowledge you. Those things and many more contributed to my success and growth in myriad ways, and I am profoundly appreciative.

To my family—my parents, sisters, brothers-in-law, and nieces and nephew—I am so grateful for the loving home I was privileged to grow up in; for Sundays on the lake, the memories of which I will always cherish; for the games we still play when we get to be together; and for the love and support I always know is there no matter what. I feel so blessed to have such an incredible family, both immediate and extended, to nurture my growth and development and help me figure out who I am.

Thanks:

Katherine Mason, Mark Sims, Marty Genereux and Julia Gumper, Leah Shearer, Alli Ward, Christine Conry, Sean Swarner, Susan Rafferty, and all those who donated money or gear or miles for making it possible for single survivors to have a meaningful adventure on the Colorado River. Twice!

Kim Wick for always reading my blog and telling me how much she got out of it.

Mike Dilbeck for insisting I join him at Author101 and getting this whole thing started!

Michelle Vos for hosting the Empowering Possibilities Summit, and all the amazing women in my "writing a book group" for encouraging me and offering advice throughout this journey.

T.J. Sullivan, Erin Weed, and Hank Nuwer for talking to me about the publishing process. Noreen Henson for finding my blog, and seeing its potential to be a book. Julia Pastore for being an incredible editor and supporter throughout the process that led to this book's publication; it is much better for her nurturing and shepherding of it.

Dwight Adkins for being the best friend anyone could ever ask for over 25 years and counting.

Pamela Graglia for always editing my blogs when I asked, and for all the great design work over the years.

Landmark Education for giving me the tools and perspective to live life powerfully and live a life that I love!

Abby and Jake Homiller for a great, quiet space on Cape Cod to complete the final edits.

The young adult cancer community for embracing my message and ME—especially Matthew Zachary, Jonny Imerman, LIVESTRONG Foundation staff, Brad Ludden, Corey Nielsen, Tamika Felder, and Marcia Donziger. I would not be where I am without you!

All the people who donated money to support me in bringing this book to life and getting it out into the world, especially: Dwight Adkins, Amy Spader, Karen Rubican, Allison Swick-Duttine, Mark Koepsell, Judy Preston, Verna Parino, Lissa and Paul Roussel, Phillip and Nancy Moye, Marcia Donziger, Drew Mann, Tim Marchell, Seana Steffen, and Marcia and Bob Maxwell. Thanks also to Give Forward for making it so easy for people to do so and for supporting the success of my campaign.

Deanne Martinez, Belinda Waldron, Wade Sheppard, and Lyna Nguyen for supporting this project, leading and coaching me to success, and holding me accountable. To all those who read drafts of the manuscript and gave me feedback which made the book better, I am truly grateful: Michelle Terhune, Darryl and Kay Armstrong, Martin Simpson, Cammie Evans, Lissa Roussel, Pamela Graglia, Marcia Donziger, Aileen Sabira Geraghty, Jeanne Johns, Christine Conry, Tommy McDowell, Ben Roussel, Cherie Michaud, Alli Ward, Jasan and Jen Zimmerman, Sage Bolte, Maureen McNamara, Leah Shearer, Judy Davidson, and Aleece Raw.

All my doctors, nurses, holistic practitioners, and health care providers who have taken such great care of me through this journey: Kathleen Tate, Daniel Donato, Sami Diab, David Gershenson, Elliott Smith, Maureen McNamara, Robyn Aasmundstad, Ban Wong, Josh Beaudry, Leigh-Erin Conneally, and all the Center For Hope staff. My amazing friends—way too numerous to list—for your tremendous support and assistance throughout this journey.

Finally, thank you to you. For what is a book without a reader?

Index

About the Author

Tracy Maxwell is the founder of Solo Survivors and The Yolo Solo, whose missions entail helping single people overcome any limiting beliefs that keep them from living lives of purpose, passion, and play. She fulfills this mission through speaking, leading programs and adventures, blogging, and coaching. Maxwell lives in Colorado, where she spends as much time as possible outside in the sunshine. Cross-country skiing is her favorite winter pastime, while river running occupies her summers as a whitewater canoe guide. During the academic year, she is often on a plane traveling to one university or another to speak to college students about hazing prevention (CAMPUSPEAK.com). This is her first book.

IamTracyMaxwell.com

About Solo Survivors

Solo Survivors began with a canoe trip in 2010 that was a project of the Self Expression and Leadership Program (SELP) through Landmark Education. Fourteen single cancer survivors from around the United States gathered to spend three days together paddling down the Colorado River. The participants ranged in age from 22 to 54, and represented different types and stages of cancer. The participants were profoundly impacted by this experience in a variety of ways.

Since then, the organization has sought new ways to support single survivors, including this book, a monthly blog, an e-mail newsletter, teleseminars, a Facebook group, and more trips and adventures. As we grow, there are plans for online and in-person gatherings (with all the tools and training for running them provided), group coaching around the concepts in the book, more teleseminars and programs, healing retreats, adventures, and trips.

Share your needs and desires with us and sign up for our mailing list at SoloSurvivors.com

About Tracy's Coaching Services

I am deeply inspired by the opportunity to coach others in identifying and releasing their limiting beliefs, recognizing their gifts, and realizing their full potential. I am a healing coach because we all have something to heal, whether it is a difficult relationship, a lack of self-confidence, a financial challenge, or a health issue. I truly believe that healing offers our best chance for creating the fulfilling lives we desire.

Healing literally means "to make whole." We are already whole, perfect, and complete, but because we don't feel that way, healing those thoughts, beliefs, patterns, traumas, and even illnesses, bring us back to a recognition of who we really are. Our identity is based on so many things, including what has happened to us, how we see the world, how we were raised, our education level, our physical appearance, our so called triumphs and failures, our family situation, what we do for a living, and so much more. We use the phrase, "I am. . ." to describe what we see as the important things about us, but the truth is, all we really need to describe us is I AM—this is our divine presence in the world, our spiritual being having a human experience.

I am especially drawn to working with other single cancer survivors, but have coached people from all backgrounds in developing more meaningful connections or creating stronger communities, negotiating new work arrangements, dealing with relationship issues or navigating a serious diagnosis. I would be thrilled to offer you a complimentary, no obligation 30 to 60 minute coaching session by phone or Skype to explore whatever challenges you are facing, and to discover how I might be able to support you.

IAmTracyMaxwell.com

Book Tracy to Speak at Your Next Conference

Tracy is an author, professional speaker, healing coach, and cancer survivor who has spoken to more than 100,000 people about changing their lives for the better. When she was diagnosed with ovarian cancer at age 36, she had no idea how she would manage as a single woman living far away from her family. In the end, Tracy's cancer diagnosis would be the catalyst for incredible improvements in her health, peace of mind, and happiness despite two recurrences and huge medical bills.

Success is due to our stretching to the challenges of life.
Failure comes when we shrink from them.
—JOHN C. MAXWELL

Tracy used her health crisis to transform her life and to help others do the same. She believes our challenges in life are what make us great. How we view the world and our environment—as friendly and supportive or hostile and unforgiving—completely determines our success in it. Tracy speaks from a place of deep compassion for what people are up against, and also insists that we take total responsibility for our own lives. Her storytelling style is inspirational, and she leaves audiences believing in their own power to create the life, love, health, and happiness that they desire.

To learn more about how to engage Tracy to talk with your group on one of many motivational topics, visit: IAmTracyMaxwell.com

About Tracy's Hazing Prevention Work

Tracy spent 20 years working in and around higher education in a variety of capacities. In this work as a consultant for her sorority, Alpha Omicron Pi, and then as a Fraternity/Sorority Advisor on a campus, she became aware of the seriousness of hazing. It wasn't something she personally experienced in her own undergraduate days, but looking back, she realized that she had experienced mild hazing in the 6th grade Beta Club, an honor society, and again as a recent college graduate during a new staff tradition at a summer camp.

But what she experienced, paled in comparison to the often brutal hazing that has caused numerous hospitalizations and even deaths. A call from an area hospital about one of her own students introduced Tracy to the fact that psychological harm from hazing was a serious problem as well, when she was told. The student had been admitted to the psych ward due to a complete mental breakdown assumed to have been brought about by the hazing he had suffered. These are the stories that are rarely told, mostly because the victims of hazing feel some measure of shame about their experience. Because the need to belong is so strong, people will do almost anything to be accepted into a group, especially one that has status, and that includes keeping quiet about the brutalities they sometimes endure as a part of that process, even when they cause serious physical or psychological harm.

Tracy founded HazingPrevention.Org, a nonprofit whose mission is to empower people to prevent hazing. She to speaks to college students about hazing through CAMPUSPEAK, www.campuspeak.com, 303-745-5545, info@campuspeak.com.